Lazy Keto Kitchen

Easy, indulgent recipes that still fit your macros

Monya Kilian Palmer

Photography by Maja Smend

KYLE BOOKS

*For all my fellow foodies, and anyone who loves being
in their kitchen as much as I love being in mine.*

An Hachette UK Company
www.hachette.co.uk

First published in Great Britain in 2021 by
Kyle Books, an imprint of Octopus Publishing Group Limited
Carmelite House
50 Victoria Embankment
London EC4Y 0DZ
www.kylebooks.co.uk

ISBN: 978-0-85783-962-6

Distributed in the US by Hachette Book Group, 1290 Avenue of the
Americas, 4th and 5th Floors, New York, NY 10104

Distributed in Canada by Canadian Manda Group, 664 Annette St.,
Toronto, Ontario, Canada M6S 2C8

Publisher: Joanna Copestick
Editorial Director: Judith Hannam
Editor: Tara O'Sullivan
Editorial Assistant: Florence Filose
Design: Nicky Collings
Photography: Maja Smend
Food Styling: Monya Kilian Palmer
Prop Styling: Morag Farquhar
Production: Lisa Pinnell

A Cataloguing in Publication record for this
title is available from the British Library

Printed and bound in China

10 9 8 7 6 5 4 3 2 1

Contents

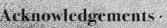

Introduction

I had so much fun creating my first book, *Keto Kitchen*, that it was inevitable a second one would soon follow. I am constantly brimming with ideas for exciting keto meals, and it is hard to stop a good thing once I get started! In fact, by the time you are reading this, it is likely I will be elbow deep in book three.

And now here you are, holding *Lazy Keto Kitchen* – another sensational labour of my love. As you will discover, I have bent the rules a little with this book, allowing for a more relaxed approach to the ketogenic lifestyle. In recent years, I discovered that many people (just like me and my husband) have never been slave to a 'macro-tracking app'. We began our journey by simply educating ourselves on which foods to avoid and which to enjoy. We kept those carbs super low and ate only when we were hungry.

I am not saying that macro-tracking apps aren't useful – many people even find them essential – I am simply saying that we never used one and we still enjoyed enormous success with the keto lifestyle. This more relaxed approach is what I understand as 'lazy keto'.

About 10–12 months into our keto journey, we realised we were eating only once a day: we had become intermittent fasters most days of the week without even planning to. However, we did (and still do) occasionally indulge in food that is popularly referred to in the 'ketosphere' as 'dirty' keto food (more on this on page 5), and this is why I wanted to put together this lazy, dirty keto cookbook. I would be a total fraud if I didn't admit to dipping my sashimi in tamari (see page 6), or including salami and pepperoni on our keto-base pizzas (for more on processed meats, see page 6).

In many cases, 'dirty' keto is unavoidable. If a friend goes to the effort of making me a lovely low-carb dinner, I am certainly not going to interrogate her on what she included in the marinade she used. And good luck to anyone holidaying in a foreign country and trying to enquire whether their steak is grass-fed or not!

Keeping carbs consistently low is core to keto if the goal is to remain in ketosis (the state where your body uses fat for fuel in the absence of carbohydrates, resulting in weight loss). To loosen up a little and have some fun in this book, though, I have unapologetically reached for convenience foods (look away now, clean-eating police!) such as pepperoni or sugar-free syrup in some recipes. I am not advising that people eat processed food all the time, because our goal is still overall health. Processed foods are considered inflammatory, and it is worth caring about what is happening inside your body on a cellular level and not only focusing on how well your jeans fit.

In the spirit of full transparency, in our home we live 'clean keto' about 85 per cent of the time. On a weekend, we may tuck into a Kielbasa Sausage Roll (page 92) made with a keto 'dough', or perhaps enjoy Garlic Pork Ribs (page 96) using a marinade made with no-added-sugar ketchup and tamari, and happily washed down with a G & sugar-free T. We remain in ketosis because the dishes are still low in carbs, albeit utterly filthy.

I try and cover the basic aspects of keto in my books, but they are first and foremost cookbooks, so I want to encourage you to delve more into the science of keto if it interests you. I have a great recommended reading list on page 143.

Every person will choose to tackle their keto journey differently, and they have a right to do what works for them. I will leave you now to page through my 'second-born'! I adore all the recipes that feature in my books, and you can be assured that if a dish did not completely smack me in the face with flavour, then it did not make the final edit. I hope you feel inspired and enjoy reading and cooking from *Lazy Keto Kitchen* as much as I enjoyed creating it!

Monya

A Keto Recap

There is so much I want to talk about in this book, so I will not repeat the finer details of keto that I covered in *Keto Kitchen*. For new readers, however, here is a brief recap.

The ketogenic lifestyle gets its name from a process in the body called ketosis. Ketosis is a very natural state for the body to be in, and it simply means a person is using fat as a fuel source as opposed to glucose from carbohydrates. The by-products of this process are called ketones, a type of chemical produced by the liver when it breaks down fat for energy. Ketones may be present in the body after periods of fasting, and in those following a ketogenic lifestyle. Remaining in this state of ketosis will (over time) result in weight loss as your body taps into fat (both stored and consumed) as its primary energy source.

As well as weight loss, those following a keto lifestyle can enjoy increased energy and mental clarity due to the reduction in blood-sugar spikes throughout the day. Blood-sugar spikes are known to leave people grumpy, hungry and fatigued. Have you ever had pasta or a large sandwich for lunch, then hit a wall at 3 p.m., ready for something sweet – or even a nap? This is because your blood sugars spike following your high-carb lunch, and then crash steeply, which leaves you hungrier and more tired than before. This does not happen on keto because your fuel source is consistent, therefore so are your energy levels.

Many people adopt a lazy, occasionally 'dirty' approach to the ketogenic lifestyle and still have plenty of weight-loss success as long as they stick to the suggested macro breakdown: very low carbs, high (natural) fat, moderate protein.

Dirty Keto

The easiest way to explain 'dirty' keto is to talk a little bit about processed food. With the keto lifestyle, there is special emphasis on eating 'clean'. This means keeping processed foods to a minimum, as they can be inflammatory to the body, playing havoc with your health over time. 'Processed food' refers to food that has been altered from its original form, often undergoing significant changes to improve flavour or extend its shelf life to make our lives more convenient.

These foods may contain additives and preservatives which our bodies could do without, which is another reason why many people choose to avoid them on keto. I would just like to tell you a little more about them and the ways in which they may – or may not – fit into your own keto lifestyle. That way, you can make the best decisions for yourself moving forward (and maybe it will help you to not be too hard on yourself if you do occasionally indulge).

It is good practice to look at the food labels when you're shopping. Not only will this enable you to calculate whether or not the carbs are worth it, you will also be able to check whether there are small amounts of gluten or some kind of sugar present, both of which are often found in low-carb products. Neither wheat nor sugar are suitable on keto, but many people sometimes 'bend' the rules because they do not have gluten intolerances or can allow for trace amounts of sugar by including them in their daily macro count. This is known as 'dirty keto'. Things like vegetable oil, alcohol and soy fall into this category.

In some of my recipes, you will notice that I call for items that may make the strict keto police shudder – I'll give you some more detail about these soon. However, I do not like to refer to my recipes as completely 'dirty', because I still care a great deal about overall health. To achieve some nutritional balance, I always make sure there are nutrient-rich ingredients present in the dishes where processed items feature, so you still get all your micro-nutrients (vitamins and minerals) while balancing your macros.

Processed Meat, Sausages & Scratchings

Delicious meats like chorizo and pepperoni are packed with flavour, as well as being low in carbs and high in fat – but it is wise to check the label, because the ingredients vary from brand to brand. Some will use only salt along with a flavouring (like smoked paprika), but some may feature a little sugar or wheat. Try to make the best decisions when selecting items like this, but it will, of course, depend on how strict you are on keto. Deli ham often features small amounts of brown sugar, while kielbasa (a smoked Polish sausage), despite being very low in carbs, contains small amounts of wheat, soy or sugar, along with several other things I cannot even pronounce. It is oh-so-delicious and packed with flavour, so it's my filthy keto pleasure.

When it comes to pork sausages, I always aim for those whose labels show they contain at least 97 per cent pork and are gluten-free. There will probably be some potato starch present, but a trace amount of potato starch in my delicious porkies (or convenient, store-bought, ready-grated mozzarella, for that matter) has never really bothered me – nor has it thrown me out of ketosis.

I usually make my own pork scratchings, but I often reach for the store-bought variety – and happily enough, my favourite brand makes a 'lean' version. Lean pork scratchings are ideal when making a keto crumb (see page 39). However, some may contain soy, wheat or dextrose (anything ending in -ose is a form of sugar).

The Gnarly Issue of Soy

I don't know about you, but I get whiplash from the information going around about soy. Medical professionals (including those doing strict keto) are telling us to avoid it like the plague due to the impact it can have on the hormones of both men and women. On the other side of the debate, there are many respected doctors telling us that we should enjoy soy and all its health benefits! I am terribly confused and have no opinion on the matter because I am not qualified to. I therefore err on the side of caution with soy: I do not consume it in large amounts (so, that's a hard no from me on tofu, tempeh and soy bean spaghetti), but when I want the delicious, rich saltiness that soy sauce offers, I reach for tamari (gluten-free soy sauce). Tamari can be found in the gluten-free aisle at stores, and most sushi restaurants will offer it as an option. If you are living clean keto or have soy allergies, you can try coconut aminos, which offers a similar flavour. I have tried it and it's lovely (although it is higher in carbs).

Konjac (Shirataki) Noodles

I love konjac products. My preferred brand comes in various shapes – the 'fettucine' and 'rice' are my favourites. These zero-carb 'noodles' are made from glucomannan fibre, which is derived from the root of the konjac plant that grows in East and Southeast Asia. They can be found in health food stores and most supermarkets. If prepared correctly, they could be a complete game-changer for you. Some may consider them 'dirty' because they are a processed food, but they contain zero carbohydrates, which means you can enjoy a decadent bowl of creamy 'pasta', 'rice' or 'risotto' guilt-free. It is also worth mentioning that glucomannan is a soluble fibre (see page 6), meaning that these products still come with some benefits. Maybe not so 'dirty' after all...

Preparing konjac (shirataki) products

There is a very funky smell present when you first open konjac products. The labels tell us to 'rinse them well', but this is not enough – more effort is required. I place them in a colander (or a large sieve if preparing the 'rice') and rinse with warm running water for several seconds, using my hand to agitate them. I go a step further by simmering them in fresh batches of water (at least 4–5 times, for several minutes each time). I promise you, the odour disappears – and the results are amazing! While I am preparing the rest of the dish, I leave the noodles (or rice) in the simmering water and drain just before using. Shirataki products will never soften like pasta or rice, but like all things in life, you get used to it. For me, it is worth the small effort, because some nights I just need to pick my battles... am I up for this 'rinse-and-repeat', or would I rather be spiralising courgettes or blitzing cauliflower?

Sugar-free Syrups

Things changed dramatically in our house after we discovered sugar-free syrups. My husband is the one with the sweet tooth, so I have gone from being a brownie-making machine (there is a beautiful brownie recipe in my first book) to having even more options with sweet treats now as I play with a range of sugar-free syrups, including flavours like 'maple' and 'salted caramel'. I refer to these syrups a handful of times in this book, but if you cannot source them in your country, you can use any sugar-free, zero-carb 'syrup'. They often contain a few unrecognisable ingredients and preservatives, which may trouble some people, but remember: they are incredibly sweet, meaning a little goes a long way.

Fats & Oils

Studies have shown that vegetable oils (like sunflower oil) or oils that oxidise easily can be highly inflammatory due to the processing they go through during production. Therefore, I threw these out years ago and do my best to avoid them as much as possible. I do, however, always have a bottle of great-quality, extra-virgin, cold-pressed olive oil in the house, which I use to finish dishes or dress salads (and would never use for frying food). To fry or stir-fry, I recommend stable fats like coconut oil, unsalted butter, lard or ghee. Ghee is an excellent option, especially for deep-frying. It is widely available, inexpensive and holds well at high temperatures. Better still, it imparts a lovely flavour!

In this book, I have called for mayonnaise in some recipes. The store-bought kind (while tasty and convenient) usually features vegetable oil, which I mentioned I try to steer clear of, so make your own (using light olive oil) if you have 10 minutes to spare. I based the macros in this book on the homemade mayonnaise recipe I shared in my first book, *Keto Kitchen*, but using store-bought should not change the macros too much.

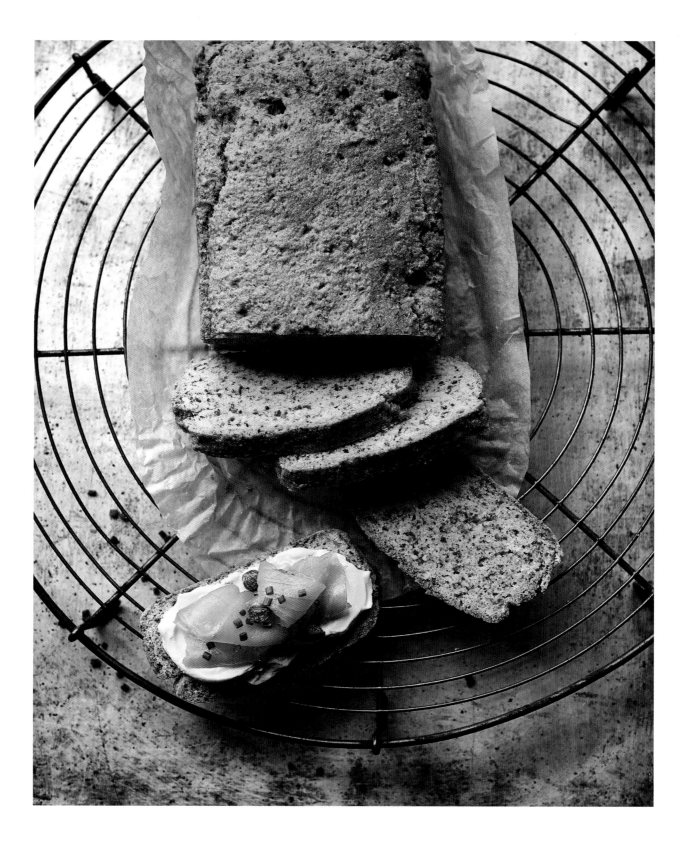

Special Ingredients

There are a handful of 'special' ingredients that I would like to address. Most of my recipes include items you can get from your local supermarket, while others can easily be sourced online.

Almond flour and coconut flour are widely available, and I find I get the best deals by buying in bulk online. However, please note the two are not interchangeable in baking; they yield different results in texture, density, and flavour. For best results, please use only what I have tried and tested.

Arrowroot powder or ground arrowroot may sound like a specialist ingredient, but it can be found right there in the baking aisle in supermarkets. I refer to it several times as it has essential thickening qualities in my recipes.

Erythritol (a sugar polyol that has no impact on blood sugar) is my preferred natural sweetener. I only use the powdered/confectioners' (not granulated) kind. Sift it before using, as some brands clump more than others. Erythritol has a slight 'cooling' effect on the palate, and I find that adding a few drops of liquid stevia balances this out. I have suggested this as an optional addition in the recipes where erythritol features in large quantities.

Ground chia seeds and ground flaxseed are sold in health food stores. Do not try and grind whole seeds yourself unless you can achieve the very fine texture the ready-ground, store-bought kinds offer. I keep all nut flours and ground seeds in a sealed container in the refrigerator to avoid possible rancidity.

Hemp seeds are a recent discovery of mine, and you will notice I use them in my Creamy Coconut Noatmeal (page 14). They are also delicious added to cauliflower rice if you want to add a little more texture and protein.

Inulin powder is a handy, store-bought soluble fibre (prebiotic) derived from chicory root. It contains only 0.4g net carbs per teaspoon, and as a supplement it is well worth the investment if this is important to you. Inulin powder is an optional addition in the Yogurt Pots (page 17), so there is no need to rush out and purchase it.

Nutritional yeast flakes are unbelievably delicious! I often stick my nose in the tub when I walk past the pantry just to take a good, long sniff because they smell heavenly! They're available everywhere and seem to be very popular with vegans, and also with vegetarians as a substitute for Parmesan cheese (which uses animal rennet). I use them in my keto-friendly crumb (see pages 39, 40 and 71).

Psyllium husk powder has fantastic thickening and binding qualities, as well as being a great source of soluble fibre. When I refer to it in my recipes, please note it is the ground powder I use. You will notice I always add it at the very end of a mixture or batter (see pages 41, 54 and 67), because it gets to work thickening the mixture very quickly. A bag will last you a long time, because only small amounts are used in any one recipe.

The Nutritional Information

The nutritional breakdown provided in this book was calculated using the cloud-based software NUTRITICS®. NUTRITICS® is fully approved by the relevant Trading Standards organisations and is EU-and FDA-compliant. I based the calculations on the trimmed weight of all the ingredients used in my recipes (apart from those shown as 'optional'). Where erythritol (see page 9) has been used, I have excluded its non-impact carbs.

Unless otherwise stated, I have shown the macro breakdown per serving, assuming the finished dish is divided into equal-sized servings. You may serve up differently, so use the nutritional information to guide your portion sizes. As I have reached for store-bought items in some recipes, you may want to double-check those, because brands differ.

Food labels vary across the world. For simplicity's sake, I have shown only the information that we monitor when eating keto: (net) carbohydrates, proteins and fats (and calories, for those who still count them).

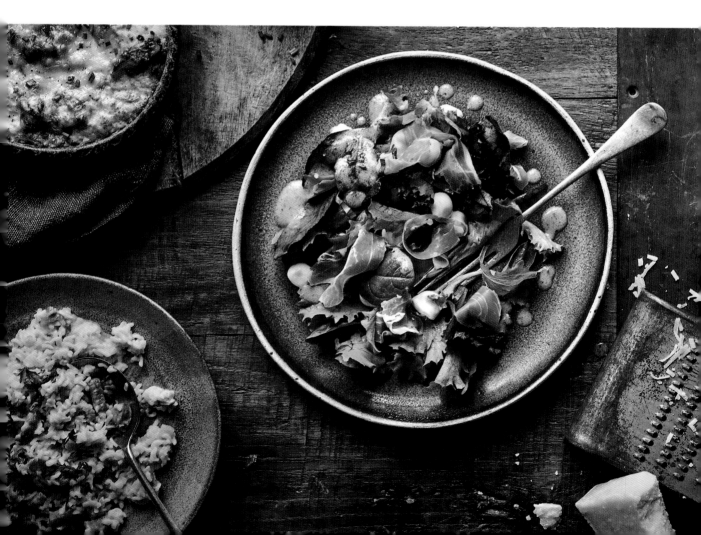

Recipe Success

- Ensure your oven is preheated before using and make sure you choose the temperature in the recipe that is given for your oven type.

- I use large eggs in the recipes, but there are two occasions where small–medium eggs are best suited, so please take note of this.

- I refer to double cream in many recipes. In the UK, this is a pourable cream with a higher fat content than regular cream. If you can't source it, use a high-fat, thickened cream and whisk it well before using to loosen it. Adding a teaspoon of water may help.

- For teaspoon or tablespoon measurements, use standard, universal measuring spoons. Dry ingredients should be levelled.

- I often add freshly chopped herbs to finish a dish after cooking. These aren't only there to make your creations more attractive – they are often essential flavour components in the recipe. The same goes for citrus elements. A squeeze of fresh lemon or lime juice offers a little acidity which can turn a good dish into a great one!

- I often mention how meat should be browned and caramelised on the outside. This is not to 'seal' the meat: that is a myth. It is simply to add additional flavour due to a chemical reaction known as the Maillard reaction. Work quickly over a high heat and do not overcrowd your pan when browning meat. Browning is best done in batches to achieve maximum caramelisation, otherwise your meat may end up simmering in its own juices, turning grey and overcooking.

- When ingredients are referred to as 'finely chopped', this means you should work your knife on them just like your favourite TV chefs do. You should aim to achieve very small pieces of approximately 3mm (⅛in) or less. Nobody wants to chew on partially cooked chunks of garlic or lemongrass, so make sure you use a good-quality, sharp knife.

- Garlic is one of my favourite ingredients! I usually add it to a pan after the onions have softened because garlic tends to burn quicker. In some recipes, where garlic is eaten raw, I suggest using a garlic press to crush the cloves effectively, getting the best texture and flavour.

- Seasoning food is important. In my recipes, I refer to salt flakes, salt, ground white pepper and freshly ground black pepper – and each have their place. When I say 'salt', I mean regular, fine salt, which I mostly use while cooking. Salt flakes should be used after cooking and only if needed. I love them because they offer little textured bursts of saltiness. When it comes to pepper, I like to use ground white pepper while cooking or in fish dishes. To finish a dish, however, a good crack of freshly ground black pepper is ideal.

- Most recipes can be made in batches and frozen, and leftovers are often even more delicious the next day. However, recipes that feature dairy (especially those using a lot of cheese, like the Cumin Flatbreads on page 110, the Cheesy 'Gnocchi' on page 112 or the Mini Rosemary Rolls on page 108) are best reheated gently in a warm oven (120°C/100°C fan/250°F/gas mark ½) for 20–25 minutes, because the microwave may not be so kind to them.

- I call for finely grated Parmesan cheese in some recipes (Pecorino or Grana Padano can also be used). I advise using the store-bought, ready-grated kind, because it is a much finer texture than you would achieve grating a block yourself. This is especially important in my keto-friendly crumb (see page 39). Plus, it is convenient – and there is nothing wrong with being a little lazy...

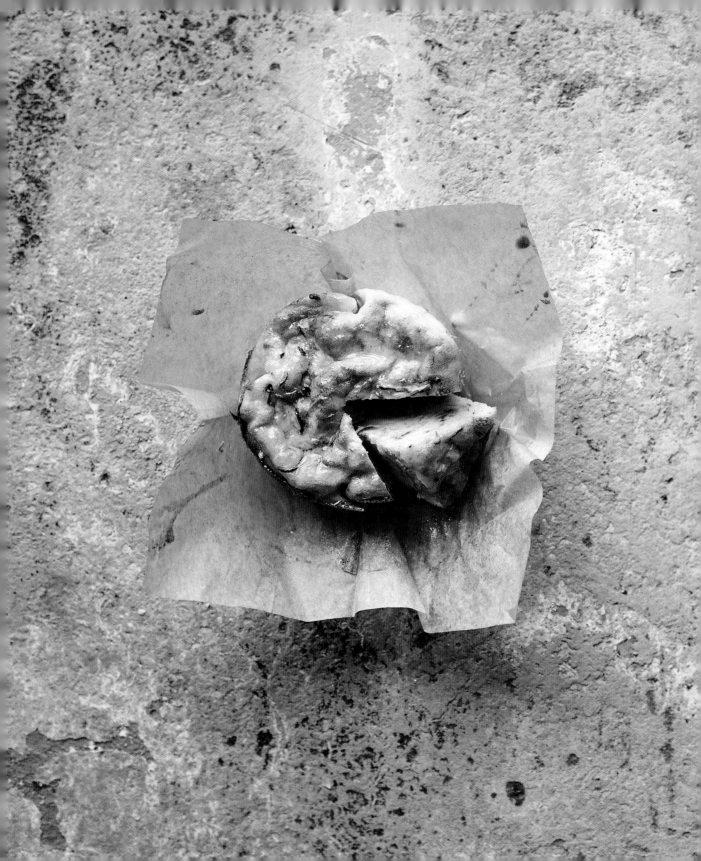

Breakfast
& Brunch

Chocolate Porridge

2 SERVINGS

10m PREP TIME

35g (1¼oz) ground flaxseed

30g (1oz) almond flour

1 tablespoon ground chia seeds

2½ tablespoons powdered erythritol, sifted

1 tablespoon unsweetened cocoa powder, sifted

250ml (9fl oz) boiling water

2–3 drops of liquid stevia (optional)

60ml (4 tablespoons) double cream

This is a fabulous, high-fibre start to the day – and who doesn't love chocolate? It is important to tuck into this porridge soon after making it, as the mixture will thicken if left standing (you don't want your entire bowl of porridge to come out with the first spoonful!).

CALORIES 358 | CARBOHYDRATES 4.1G | PROTEIN 9G | FAT 32G

Place the ground flaxseed, almond flour and ground chia seeds in a bowl. Stir through the erythritol and cocoa powder. Add the boiling water and mix well to combine. Add a few drops of liquid stevia (if using) and divide between 2 bowls. Enjoy immediately, drizzled with the double cream.

Creamy Coconut Noatmeal

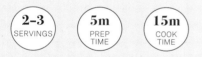

2–3 SERVINGS

5m PREP TIME

15m COOK TIME

400g (14oz) can full-fat coconut milk

40g (1½oz) desiccated coconut

2 tablespoons coconut flour

45g (1½oz) shelled hemp seeds

2 tablespoons powdered erythritol, sifted

This lovely bowl of goodness features hemp seeds, which give plenty of 'body' to this hearty breakfast. It can be enjoyed any time of the day (as a teenager I would often eat porridge on a Sunday night). The macros are calculated on a cooked serving of 140g (5oz), excluding toppings.

CALORIES 516 | CARBOHYDRATES 9.4G | PROTEIN 9.3G | FAT 48G

Shake the can of coconut milk well before opening, then pour the contents into a medium-sized saucepan. Bring to a simmer, then add all the remaining ingredients, stirring well to combine. Cook the mixture for 10–12 minutes or until the coconut milk reduces by half and you are left with a thick, porridge-like consistency. Divide between serving bowls and serve topped with fresh berries (if your macros allow for it).

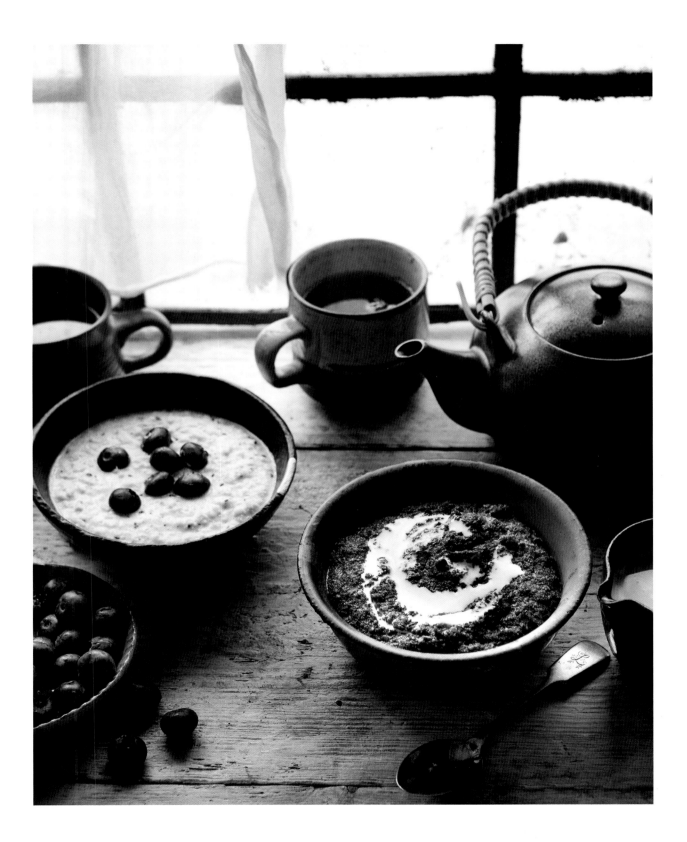

Double Creamy Coffee

1 SERVING   **5m** PREP TIME

40ml (1¼fl oz) double cream

1 tablespoon collagen protein powder

1 teaspoon MCT oil (see Tip)

your chosen sweetener (if using)

1 serving of hot black coffee (or coffee pod, if you use a machine)

This is my favourite way to drink coffee. It is so rich and filling, and can satiate you for many hours. The most important thing is that the fats are emulsified in the hot coffee. Some people use butter or coconut oil in place of cream (which is equally delicious). *Pictured on page 19.*

CALORIES 259 | CARBOHYDRATES 0.6G | PROTEIN 8G | FAT 25G

Place the cream, collagen powder and MCT oil in your coffee mug. If you like sweet coffee (like I do), add the sweetener now, too. Use a mini whisk to combine the mixture well. Place your mug under your coffee machine and pop in the pod, or pour over a prepared cup of hot black coffee. Give it one more thorough whisk before enjoying.

- MCT oil is an excellent energy source and promotes a feeling of fullness. Over time, you can gradually increase the MCT oil to 1 tablespoon.
- Collagen can contribute to the maintenance of skin and joints. It is also a great way to increase your protein intake.

Cinnamon Flax Breakfast Muffins

9 MUFFINS   **15m** PREP TIME   **25m** COOK TIME

4 large eggs

100g (3½oz) soured cream

4–5 drops of liquid stevia (optional)

80g (2¾oz) unflavoured coconut oil, melted and cooled a little

For the 'dry mix'

150g (5½oz) almond flour

110g (3¾oz) powdered erythritol, sifted

45g (1½oz) ground flaxseed

1 teaspoon baking powder

1 teaspoon bicarbonate of soda

2 tablespoons ground cinnamon

Not only are these muffins high in fibre (thank you, ground flaxseed), they are also super tasty! They freeze well, too, so make a great back-up snack option. Try adding some roughly chopped nuts to the mix before baking, for a lovely crunchy texture. *Pictured on page 19.*

CALORIES 272 | CARBOHYDRATES 3.5G | PROTEIN 8G | FAT 24G

Preheat the oven to 180°C/160°C fan/350°F/gas mark 4 and line a muffin tray with 9 paper cases.

In a bowl, whisk together the eggs, soured cream and liquid stevia (if using), then whisk in the cooled melted coconut oil.

Combine all the 'dry' ingredients in a separate bowl, ensuring they are evenly mixed. Pour the wet mixture into the flour mixture and stir well to combine. Divide the mixture evenly between the paper cases, filling them half to three-quarters full.

Bake for 10 minutes, then reduce the oven temperature to 160°C/140°C fan/325°F/gas mark 3 and bake for an additional 15 minutes, or until a skewer inserted into the centre of a muffin comes out clean. Remove from the tin and leave to cool on a wire rack before serving.

Yogurt Pots
with 'Maple' Syrup

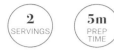

We love a little bowl of yogurt and berries, and my husband Mark often enjoys this as a quick dessert on the nights when no other treats are kicking about. The inulin powder is optional, but a fantastic way to increase prebiotics in the diet (see page 6). *Pictured on page 18.*

CALORIES 128 | CARBOHYDRATES 7.1G | PROTEIN 5G | FAT 8.3G

2 SERVINGS   **5m** PREP TIME

160g (5¾oz) full-fat plain yogurt

2 teaspoons inulin powder (optional)

90g (3¼oz) mixed berries (I used equal amounts blackberries, blueberries and raspberries for varying sweetness and acidity)

2 teaspoons sugar-free 'maple' syrup

Place the yogurt in a bowl and stir in the inulin powder (if using). Fold through the berries, then divide the mixture between 2 small breakfast bowls. Drizzle over the sugar-free 'maple' syrup and tuck in!

Rolled Crêpes
with Cinnamon 'Sugar'

Growing up, we always ate crêpes with a generous sprinkle of cinnamon sugar, so I've made a version with erythritol. These delicate crêpes are best made in a good-quality, non-stick frying pan that is completely free of rust and scratches. *Pictured on page 18.*

CALORIES 181 | CARBOHYDRATES 2G | PROTEIN 5G | FAT 17G

9–10 CRÊPES   **20m** PREP TIME   **30m** COOK TIME

100g (3½oz) full-fat cream cheese

4 large eggs

70g (2½oz) almond flour

3 tablespoons powdered erythritol, sifted

2–3 drops of liquid stevia (optional)

145ml (5fl oz) double cream

2 tablespoons unflavoured coconut oil, melted

sugar-free 'maple' syrup, to serve (optional)

For the cinnamon 'sugar'

2 tablespoons powdered erythritol, sifted

2 teaspoons ground cinnamon

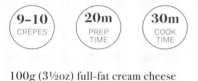

In a bowl, use a hand blender to blitz together the cream cheese, eggs, almond flour, erythritol and liquid stevia (if using) until smooth and free of lumps. Switch to using a whisk and whisk in the double cream. In a separate bowl, combine the cinnamon 'sugar' ingredients.

Place a large non-stick frying pan over a medium heat and lightly grease with a little melted coconut oil. Pour 60ml (4 tablespoons) batter into the pan and swirl so the mixture coats the bottom in a thin layer. Cook for 2–2½ minutes, then quickly – but carefully! – flip it over. Cook on the other side for 1 minute, then set aside on a plate, sprinkling with the cinnamon 'sugar' before rolling up.

Repeat for the remaining crêpes, wiping the pan with a little more coconut oil each time. Scatter any leftover cinnamon 'sugar' over the top before serving. Serve with sugar-free 'maple' syrup, if you like.

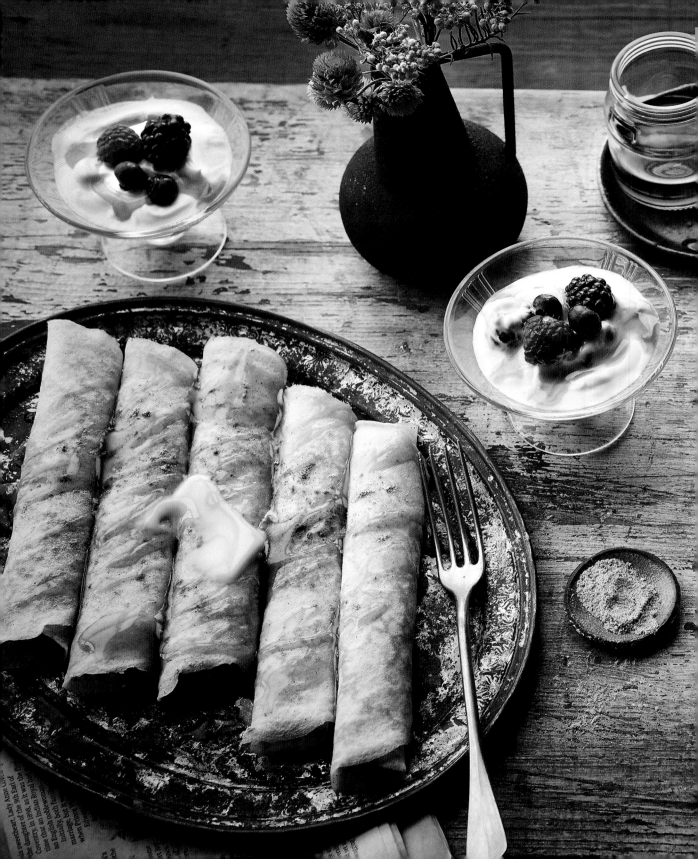

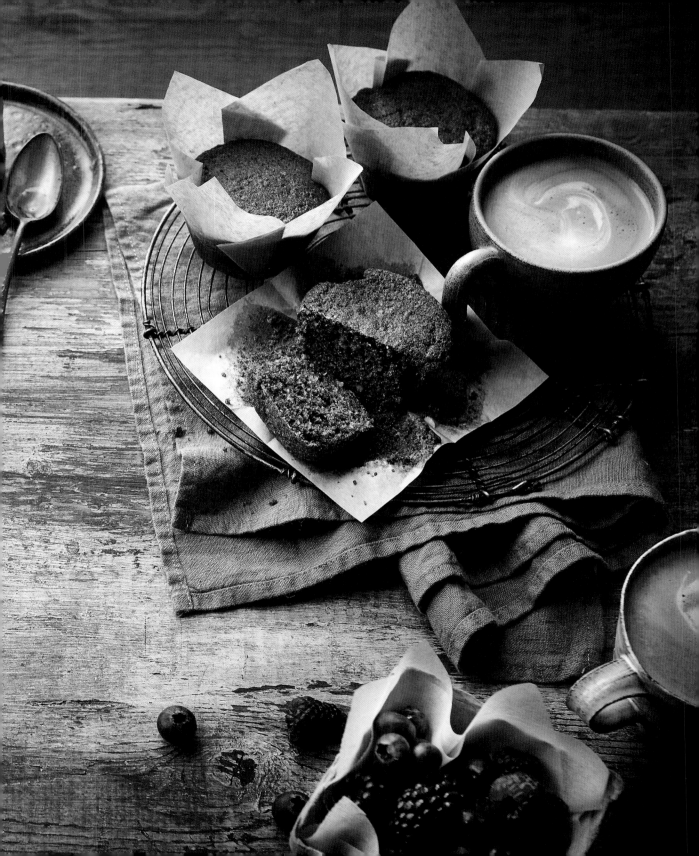

Pepperoni Egg Bake

You will love this rich, filling little dish. Although I've put it in the breakfast section, we often have it at dinner time with a fresh green salad on the side. I used spicy pepperoni here, but thin slices of any full-flavoured deli meat (like salami) would work equally well. If you do not have small, shallow dishes as shown, you can prepare this in ramekins, but you may need to increase the cooking time slightly to ensure the eggs are cooked through. Here, both the yolks and whites will set; this is normal.

CALORIES 487 | CARBOHYDRATES 1.1G | PROTEIN 19G | FAT 45G

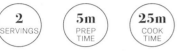

2 SERVINGS | 5m PREP TIME | 25m COOK TIME

120ml (4fl oz) double cream

4 large eggs

20g (¾oz) pepperoni slices, chopped into smaller pieces

salt flakes, salt, ground white pepper and freshly ground black pepper

freshly chopped chives, to garnish

Preheat the oven to 200°C/180°C fan/400°F/gas mark 6.

Take 2 shallow ovenproof dishes, approximately 10 x 15cm (4 x 6in), and pour about 40ml (1¼fl oz) double cream into each.

Crack 2 eggs into each dish, being careful not to break the yolks. Cover with the remaining cream and season with salt and ground white pepper. Scatter the chopped pepperoni pieces into the cream.

Place the dishes on a baking tray (for easier removal) and bake for 20 minutes, or until the mixture has set. If you are using ramekins instead, you may need to add another 5 minutes to the cooking time.

Season with a few salt flakes (only if needed) and some freshly ground black pepper. Scatter over the fresh chives and tuck in!

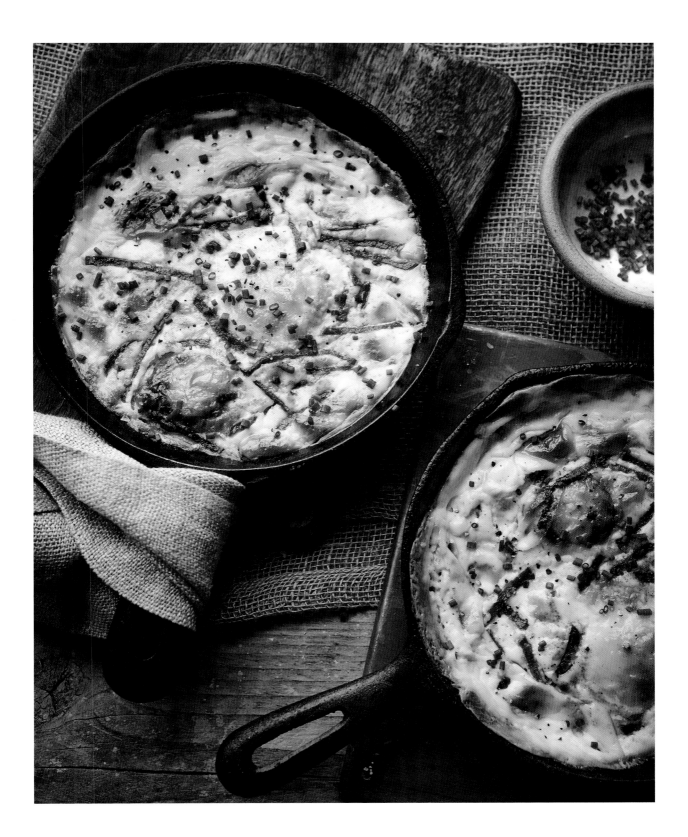

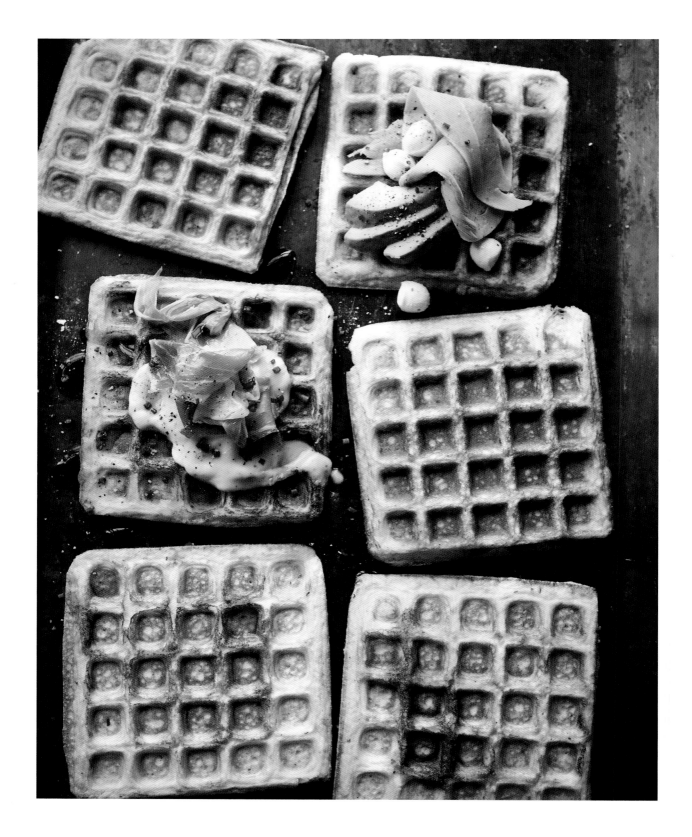

Savoury Waffles

2 SERVINGS | **10m** PREP TIME | **10m** COOK TIME

4 large eggs

110g (3¾oz) flavoured cream cheese

25g (1oz) almond flour

1 teaspoon baking powder

salt and freshly ground black pepper

toppings/garnishes of your choice

Waffles do not always need to be sweet! These are made using a flavoured cream cheese, but the best part is that you can have some fun with your toppings. This recipe makes two waffles (in my waffle maker), and the macros shown are per waffle, excluding any toppings.

PER WAFFLE | CALORIES 310 | CARBOHYDRATES 5.5G | PROTEIN 21G | FAT 22G

Whisk together the eggs and cream cheese in a bowl. In a separate bowl, combine the almond flour and baking powder. Add this dry mix to the eggs and whisk very well to create a smooth batter with no lumps. Season generously with salt and freshly ground black pepper.

Grease and preheat your waffle maker according to the manufacturer's instructions, then pour in the batter and cook until done. Opening the waffle maker too soon can ruin them; I always open mine about 1 minute after it tells me they are ready. Remove the waffles and enjoy. You could simply serve with melted butter and a scattering of salt flakes or herbs, but I love them with mozzarella and prosciutto. You could also try avocado and ham, or crispy bacon and no-added-sugar ketchup.

Cheesy Courgette Egg 'Muffins'

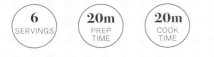

6 SERVINGS | **20m** PREP TIME | **20m** COOK TIME

300g (10½oz) courgettes, grated and squeezed until dry (see Tip on page 25; weight given is before squeezing)

60g (2¼oz) extra-mature full-fat Cheddar cheese, finely grated

4 large eggs

100ml (3½fl oz) double cream

1 teaspoon baking powder

salt and ground white pepper

Ridiculously yummy and so, so rich. These little muffins are packed with grated courgette, and the flavour is fresh and wonderful! They can be stored in the refrigerator – just a few seconds in the microwave will bring them back to life. They freeze well, too. *Pictured on page 12.*

CALORIES 182 | CARBOHYDRATES 1.9G | PROTEIN 8.4G | FAT 15G

Preheat the oven to 200°C/180°C fan/400°F/gas mark 6 and line a muffin tray with 6 paper muffin cases.

Place the grated, squeezed courgettes in a bowl and stir in the Cheddar.

In a separate bowl, whisk together the eggs and double cream. Sift in the baking powder and whisk well to combine. Pour the egg mixture into the cheesy courgette mixture and season before stirring well.

Divide the mixture evenly between the paper cases, filling them halfway to three-quarters full. Bake for 20 minutes, then remove from the oven and allow to cool slightly before enjoying.

Breakfast Towers

with Swede Hash Browns

I came up with this great method for cooking swede 'hash browns' by doing everything in reverse to ensure they do not fall apart. I bake them first so that the mixture sets, then lightly fry them to achieve the lovely caramelisation. This is a generous breakfast tower that will dazzle your house guests on a morning when you are feeling ambitious!

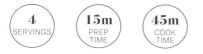

4 SERVINGS | 15m PREP TIME | 45m COOK TIME

CALORIES 434 | CARBOHYDRATES 9.4G | PROTEIN 23G | FAT 33G

3 tablespoons unsalted butter

200g (7oz) smoked bacon lardons

240g (8½oz) baby spinach

2 tablespoons soured cream

1 tablespoon white vinegar

4 large eggs

2 tomatoes, sliced into 8 even slices

freshly ground black pepper

freshly chopped chives, to garnish

For the swede hash browns

500g (1lb 2oz) swede, peeled, grated and squeezed until dry (see Tip; weight given is before squeezing)

20g (¾oz) Parmesan cheese, finely grated

3 spring onions, very finely chopped

1 large egg, whisked

pinch of paprika

salt and ground white pepper

Preheat the oven to 160°C/140°C fan/325°F/gas mark 3.

Begin by making the hash browns. Place the grated, squeezed swede in a bowl and stir through the Parmesan and spring onions. Add the whisked egg and season with paprika, salt and ground white pepper.

Divide into 8 even-sized portions and place on a baking tray lined with baking paper. Neaten into little 'patties'. Bake on the lowest rack of the oven for 25–30 minutes, rotating the tray halfway through.

Meanwhile, heat 1 tablespoon of the butter in a large non-stick frying pan and cook the bacon lardons for 5–10 minutes until cooked through. Remove using a slotted spoon, leaving all the juices in the pan, and set aside. Add the spinach to the pan and cook until wilted. Stir through the soured cream and return the bacon to the pan. Season with black pepper and stir, then transfer to a bowl and keep warm.

Add the remaining butter to the frying pan. Gently remove the hash browns from the baking tray and fry them in the butter until browned and crispy on both sides. Set aside to keep warm.

Bring a large saucepan of water to the boil over a medium heat and add the vinegar. Reduce the heat to a low simmer and stir the water to create a swirl. Crack in 2 of the eggs and poach for 3–4 minutes before removing with a slotted spoon and placing on a plate lined with paper towels. Repeat with the other 2 eggs.

To assemble, divide the bacon-and-spinach mixture between 4 plates. Layer the swede hash browns and sliced tomatoes on top, then finish each tower with a poached egg. Season, and scatter over the chives before serving.

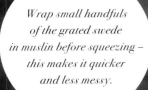

*

Wrap small handfuls of the grated swede in muslin before squeezing – this makes it quicker and less messy.

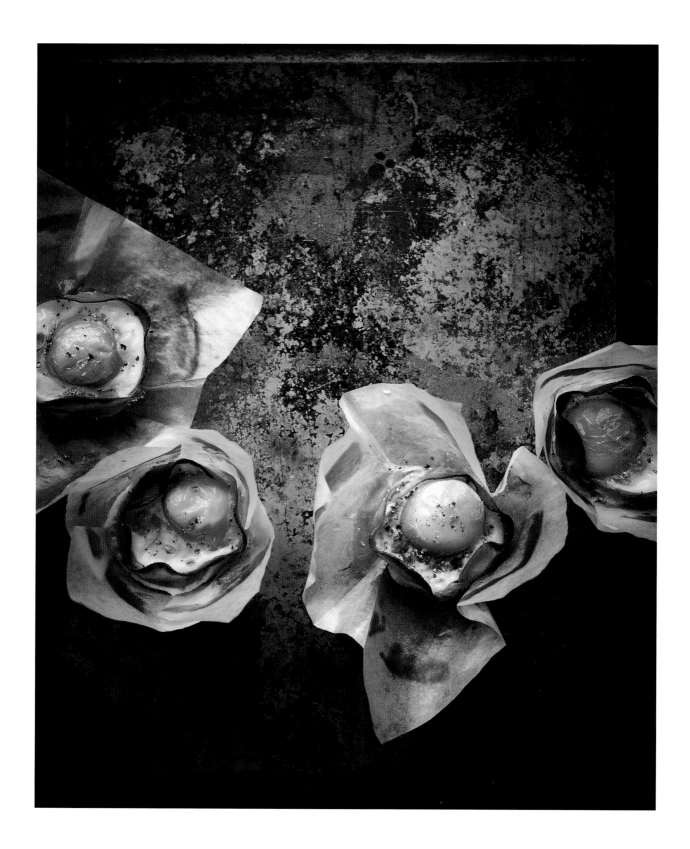

Ham & Mushroom Egg Cups

These are a fun way to enjoy a rich breakfast made using eggs and ham. The star of the show, however, is the unseen layer tucked in under the eggs, which features a thyme-flavoured caramelised mushroom mixture. You will notice I use small–medium eggs for this specific recipe, as larger ones would cause the little cases to overflow.

6 SERVINGS | **15m** PREP TIME | **25m** COOK TIME

CALORIES 123 | CARBOHYDRATES 1.3G | PROTEIN 11G | FAT 8.4G

1 tablespoon unsalted butter

100g (3½oz) mushrooms, finely chopped

4 fresh thyme sprigs, leaves picked

30g (1oz) extra-mature full-fat Cheddar cheese, finely grated

6 slices of deli ham (approx. 100g/3½oz total)

6 small–medium eggs

salt flakes, salt, ground white pepper and freshly ground black pepper

Preheat the oven to 200°C/180°C fan/400°F/gas mark 6 and line a muffin tray with 6 paper cases.

Melt the butter in a non-stick frying pan over a medium heat and cook the mushrooms until they have completely softened and caramelised, and there is no moisture left in the pan. Remove from the heat and stir through the thyme leaves and grated cheese. Season with salt and ground white pepper, then set aside.

Cut out 2 small triangles from the top and bottom of each slice of ham – this makes it easier to fold it in on itself, forming a little round 'cup' which will not leak. Place each ham 'cup' inside a paper case. Divide the cheesy mushroom mixture between the 6 ham 'cups' and press down to compress. Crack an egg into each one, then bake for 15–18 minutes, rotating the muffin tray halfway through to ensure even cooking, until the egg whites are opaque.

Remove from the muffin tray and serve with salt flakes (if needed) and a crack of black pepper.

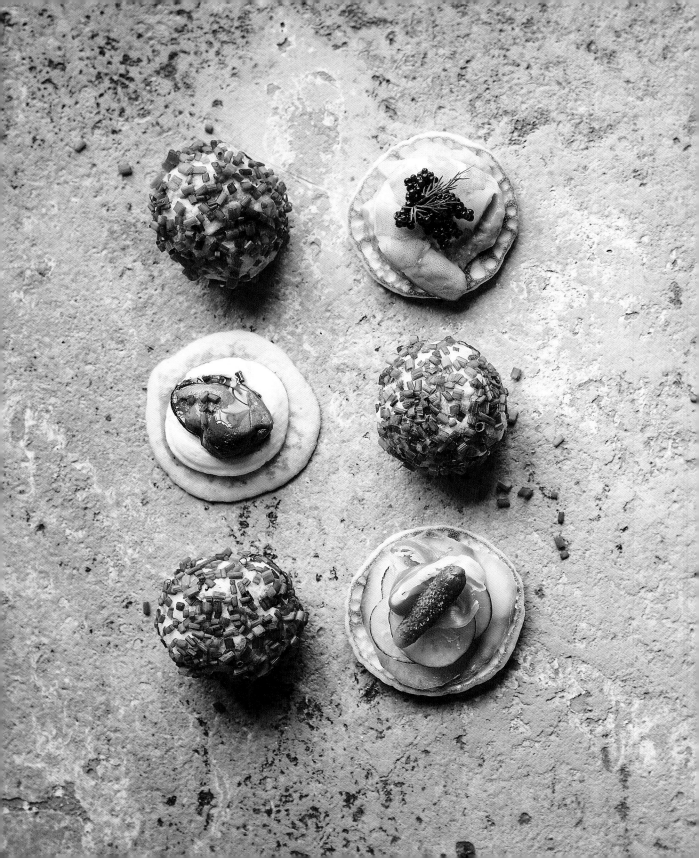

Tapas &
Small Bites

Caraway & Flax Crackers

Deliciously crispy with a lovely caraway flavour, these crackers are ideal for scooping up guacamole or any of your favourite keto dips. I love to serve them with a Baked Camembert (page 37), as pictured. After the first bake, you can slice them into any shape you choose, but I like to make seven long crackers, and that's what the macros here are based on. If you aren't a fan of caraway, replace the caraway seeds with 4 tablespoons nutritional yeast flakes for a 'cheesier' flavour, or 3 tablespoons mixed seeds for seedy crackers bursting with goodness!

7 SERVINGS   **10m** PREP TIME   **20m** COOK TIME

CALORIES 89 | CARBOHYDRATES 1.7G | PROTEIN 4.6G | FAT 6.5G

35g (1¼oz) almond flour

3 tablespoons ground flaxseed

½ teaspoon salt

¼ teaspoon garlic powder

¼ teaspoon mustard powder

3 tablespoons caraway seeds, ground lightly in a pestle and mortar

2 large eggs, very well whisked

salt flakes

*

If you find the crackers lose their crispness, simply pop them into a warm oven (or even an air fryer on the dehydrator setting) for a few minutes.

Preheat the oven to 220°C/200°C fan/425°F/gas mark 7 and place a silicone mat on a large baking tray. Cut a large sheet of baking paper and set aside for later.

In a bowl, mix together the almond flour, ground flaxseed, salt, garlic powder, mustard powder and lightly ground caraway seeds.

Pour in the whisked eggs and mix well to combine. Tip the mixture out on to the silicone baking mat and use a silicone spatula to spread it out into a rectangle measuring approximately 21 x 30cm (8¼ x 12in). It should be thin, but without any holes – it will feel a little like you are plastering a wall! Neaten the edges and scatter over some salt flakes.

Bake for just 6 minutes on the lowest shelf, then remove the tray from the oven. Here is the tricky part: place the sheet of baking paper on top of the partially baked mixture and very gently flip the entire thing so that you can bake the underside. I find that the easiest way of doing this is to place a second large baking tray on top, then quickly flip it.

Your partially baked mixture will now have the baking paper underneath it, and you will no longer need the silicone mat. Use a pizza cutter to slice it into crackers in the size and shape of your choice. The 'dough' should not have cooked too hard yet, so will be easy to slice.

Return the tray to the oven for an additional 8–9 minutes. When you take it out, you will notice the crackers have hardened. If you want more colour, flip each cracker and return to the oven until you are happy with their crispness and colour. Place the crackers on a wire rack to cool completely, then store in a sealed container, where they will keep for up to 1 week.

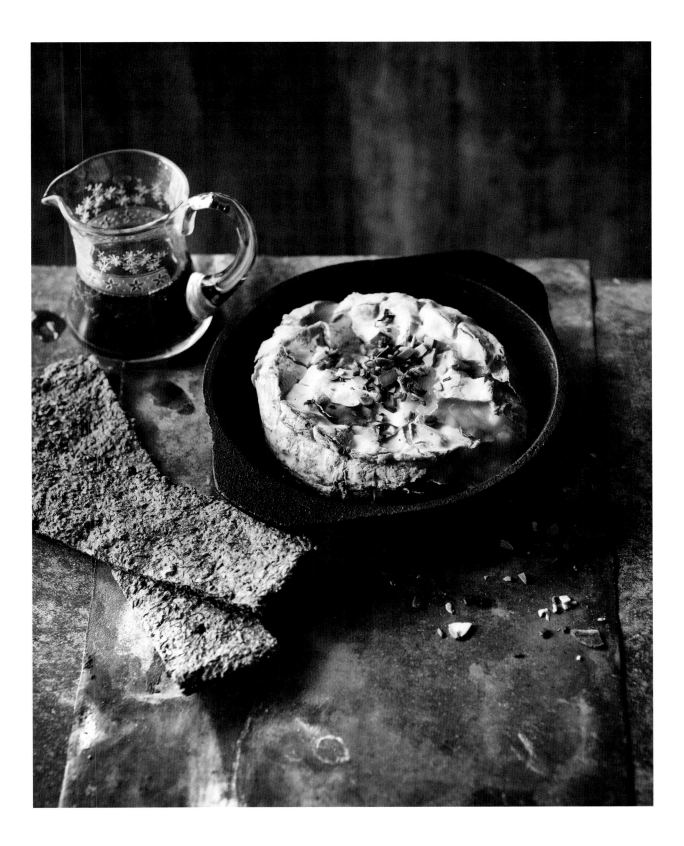

Spicy Cheese Crackers

with Dynamite Salsa

This is an easy little appetiser to put out for guests at your next *braai* (barbecue) – and it could not be simpler! Be sure to use a mild, ready-sliced cheese (I like Edam) and follow the oven times and temperatures exactly as indicated. The fresh tomato and chilli salsa perfectly complements the cheesy flavour of the crackers. The macros are calculated on this recipe (crackers and salsa) being shared between four people.

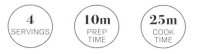

4 SERVINGS | **10m** PREP TIME | **25m** COOK TIME

CALORIES 209 | CARBOHYDRATES 2.3G | PROTEIN 16G | FAT 14G

For the crackers

10 slices of mild cheese (e.g. Edam, approx. 250g/9oz total)

pinch of smoked paprika

pinch of cayenne pepper

For the salsa

2 tomatoes, finely chopped

½ small red onion, finely chopped

1 small red chilli, finely chopped

juice of ½ lime

small handful of fresh coriander leaves, finely chopped

Preheat the oven to 220°C/200°C fan/425°F/gas mark 7 and line a baking tray with baking paper or a silicone mat.

Slice each cheese slice into 4 smaller triangles and place them on the lined tray, leaving a little space between each piece, as they may spread slightly. You may need to cook them in 2 or 3 batches depending on the size of your tray, but fear not – it won't take long.

Cook for exactly 8 minutes, rotating the tray halfway through. Remove from the oven and wait a minute or two, then gently remove each cracker from the tray using a small silicone spatula. Place on a wire rack to cool – they will crisp up as they cool.

To make the salsa, place the tomatoes, onion and chilli in a bowl and stir to combine. Squeeze over the lime juice and stir through the chopped coriander.

Serve the crackers with the salsa.

If you're not eating the crackers right away, they can be stored in a sealed container at room temperature for 1–2 days. To crisp them up, lay out on a lined baking tray and bake for 3–4 minutes at 140°C/120°C fan/275°F/gas mark 1.

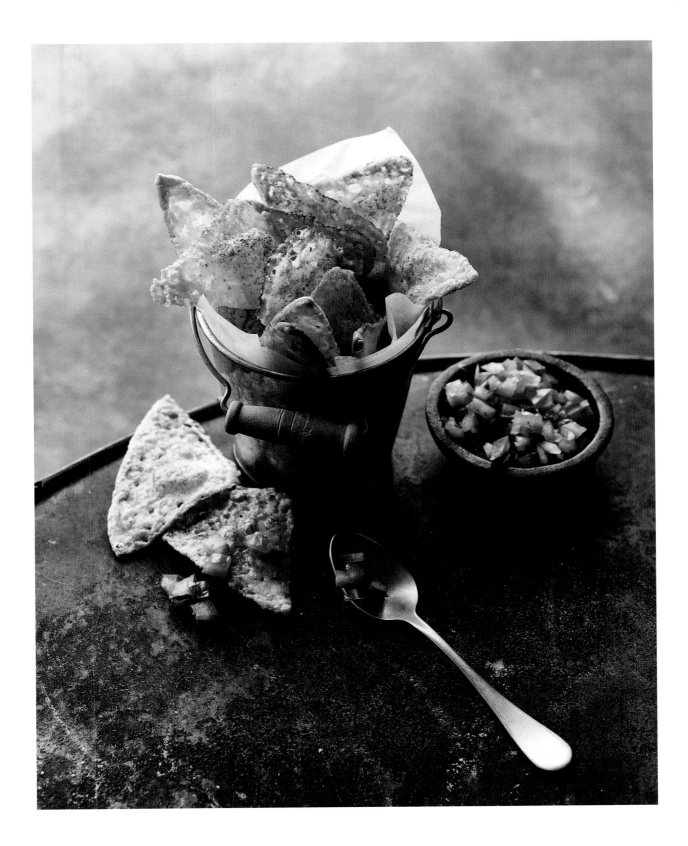

Ham & Gruyère Pinwheel Rolls

I posted a photo of myself tucking into my recipe trial of these rolls on Instagram and it was so well-received, I simply had to perfect the recipe so that I could share it far and wide. Once you've mastered the method, you can have some fun by changing up the fillings: why not try sliced salami and crumbled feta, or basil pesto and grated Cheddar? More importantly, do not be too hard on yourself if your rolls end up looking a little rustic and imperfect. Most things made with love do.

4 ROLLS | **15m** PREP TIME | **45m** CHILL TIME | **25m** COOK TIME

CALORIES 457 | CARBOHYDRATES 3.9G | PROTEIN 29G | FAT 36G

100g (3½oz) almond flour

1 teaspoon baking powder

1 teaspoon garlic powder

pinch of salt

100g (3½oz) grated mozzarella cheese

60g (2¼oz) full-fat cream cheese

130g (4¾oz) Gruyère cheese, grated

1 large egg, very well whisked

120g (4¼oz) sliced deli ham (approx. 7 slices)

Preheat the oven to 200°C/180°C fan/400°F/gas mark 6.

In a bowl, mix together the almond flour, baking powder, garlic powder and salt, then transfer to a mini food processor. In a second, wide-bottomed bowl, mix the grated mozzarella with the cream cheese and 70g (2½oz) of the Gruyère.

Place the bowl of cheese in the microwave on high for 60–90 seconds until melted. Tip the melted cheese into the food processor containing the dry ingredients and blitz well. Add the whisked egg and continue to mix until the mixture comes together to form a sticky dough.

Tip the dough out on to a long sheet of baking paper and cover with a second sheet. Use a rolling pin to roll out the dough into a long rectangle measuring approximately 18 x 30cm (7 x 12in). Slide on to a baking tray and place in the refrigerator for 45 minutes to firm up a little.

Peel away the top sheet of baking paper. Neaten up the edges of the rectangle. Lay the slices of ham on top of the dough and sprinkle over the remaining Gruyère. Gently roll up the dough, starting with one of the shorter sides, to create a fat log. Hold a sharp knife under very hot running water, then use it to slice the cylinder into 4 equal-sized pieces, running the knife under hot water again between each slice.

Place the pieces, cut-side up, in a small baking tray lined with baking paper. Bake for 20 minutes, then turn off the oven and leave the rolls in there to finish baking in the residual heat for another 5 minutes before removing and enjoying while still warm.

*

The chilled dough should be quite manageable, but if you encounter any 'holes' as you're rolling up the log, you can pinch them closed.

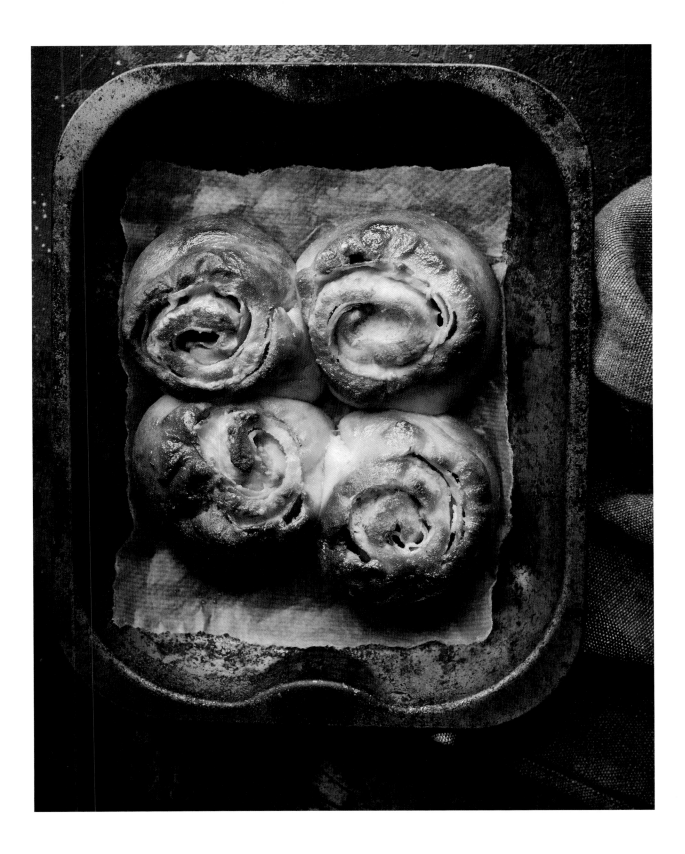

'Afternoon Tea' Mini Loaf

(**1** SMALL LOAF) (**10m** PREP TIME) (**35m** COOK TIME)

50g (1¾oz) unsalted butter

3 large eggs, whisked

150g (5½oz) almond flour

3 tablespoons ground chia seeds

1½ teaspoons baking powder

½ teaspoon salt

2 teaspoons psyllium husk powder

This lovely textured loaf yields 10–12 slices. It's perfect for making little open sandwiches for a keto afternoon tea, perhaps with cream cheese and smoked salmon, or roast beef, cornichons and mustard. Macros are calculated per slice, excluding toppings. *Pictured on page 8.*

PER SLICE: CALORIES 139 | CARBOHYDRATES 1.3G | PROTEIN 4.9G | FAT 12G

Preheat the oven to 200°C/180°C fan/400°F/gas mark 6 and line a 900g (2lb) loaf tin with baking paper or a loaf liner.

Melt the butter in a saucepan over a medium–high heat and allow it to foam. You will notice a nutty smell as the milk solids brown. Remove from the heat and allow to cool slightly, then pour into a bowl with the eggs and whisk. In a separate bowl, mix together all the remaining ingredients. Pour the egg mixture into the dry mixture and mix well, then transfer to the prepared loaf tin. Bake for 25 minutes, then turn off the oven and leave the loaf inside for an additional 5 minutes, or until a skewer inserted into the centre comes out clean. Remove from the oven and allow to cool completely on a wire rack.

Bacon & Chive Fat Bombs

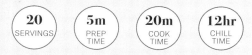

(**20** SERVINGS) (**5m** PREP TIME) (**20m** COOK TIME) (**12hr** CHILL TIME)

125g (4½oz) unsalted butter

380g (13½oz) smoked streaky bacon, finely chopped

4 garlic cloves, finely chopped

100g (3½oz) full-fat cream cheese

50g (1¾oz) soured cream

10g (¼oz) freshly chopped chives (plus an extra 10g/¼oz to coat, optional)

freshly ground black pepper

I rarely feel truly hungry (high five to the keto lifestyle!), but I do still enjoy a bite-sized, full-flavoured fatty snack in the late afternoon to satiate me until dinner time. Keep a few of these delicious bombs in the refrigerator for an easy grab-and-go option. *Pictured on page 28.*

CALORIES 133 | CARBOHYDRATES 0.6G | PROTEIN 5.6G | FAT 12G

Melt the butter in a large non-stick frying pan over a medium heat. Add the bacon and garlic and cook for 15–20 minutes, stirring regularly. It is important that all excess juice and moisture is cooked out and you are left with only fat. Remove the pan from the heat and stir in the cream cheese and soured cream, along with the 10g (¼oz) chives. Season with black pepper and mix well. Transfer to a large bowl and chill overnight to allow all the fat to solidify completely.

The next day, form the solidified mixture into 20 smooth balls of approximately 27g (1oz) each – an ice-cream scoop is best for this. If you like, you can roll them in chives, to coat. They will keep in the refrigerator for 3–4 days, but they freeze well, too.

Baked Camembert
with Sugar-free 'Maple' Syrup & Almonds

4 SERVINGS · 5m PREP TIME · 25m COOK TIME

250g (9oz) best-quality Camembert round (for best results, remove from the refrigerator 30 minutes before baking)

10g (¼oz) flaked almonds

1 tablespoon sugar-free 'maple' syrup

freshly chopped chives, to garnish (optional)

Deliciously oozy, this simple baked Camembert is a fabulous option when entertaining friends, and perfect scooped up with my Caraway & Flax Crackers (page 30). Enjoy the simple indulgence! *Pictured on page 31.*

CALORIES 185 | CARBOHYDRATES 0.8G | PROTEIN 14G | FAT 14G

Preheat the oven to 200°C/180°C fan/400°F/gas mark 6.

Place the Camembert in a suitable ovenproof dish (or a Camembert baker, if you have one) and bake for 20–25 minutes.

Meanwhile, toast the flaked almonds in a dry non-stick pan over a medium heat until golden. Once toasted, roughly chop.

To serve, drizzle the sugar-free 'maple' syrup over the oozy baked Camembert and scatter over the almonds. Finish with chopped chives if you are feeling fancy.

Blinis!

40 BLINIS · 10m PREP TIME · 30m COOK TIME

50g (1¾oz) full-fat cream cheese

2 large eggs

45g (1½oz) almond flour

½ teaspoon baking powder

65ml (2¼fl oz) double cream

2 tablespoons unflavoured coconut oil, melted

salt and ground white pepper

These blinis are ideal for parties. Get creative with toppings – I love crème fraîche and smoked mussels! Macros are based on two blinis, excluding toppings. Be sure to use a good-quality, non-stick frying pan that is completely free of rust and scratches. *Pictured on page 28.*

CALORIES 50 | CARBOHYDRATES 0.5G | PROTEIN 1.4G | FAT 4.8G

Place the cream cheese, eggs and almond flour in a small jug or bowl. Sift in the baking powder, then use a hand blender to blitz into a smooth batter, free of lumps. Season with salt and ground white pepper. Switch to using a whisk and lightly whisk in the double cream.

Place a large non-stick frying pan over a medium heat and lightly grease with a little melted coconut oil. Working in batches of 4 at a time, drop in ½ tablespoon batter for each blini. Leave for 2 minutes, and you will notice little bubbles appearing. Use a small silicone spatula to gently lift and turn the blinis, cooking the underside for about 45–50 seconds. Set aside on a plate before repeating the process until all the blinis are made. Serve with your choice of toppings.

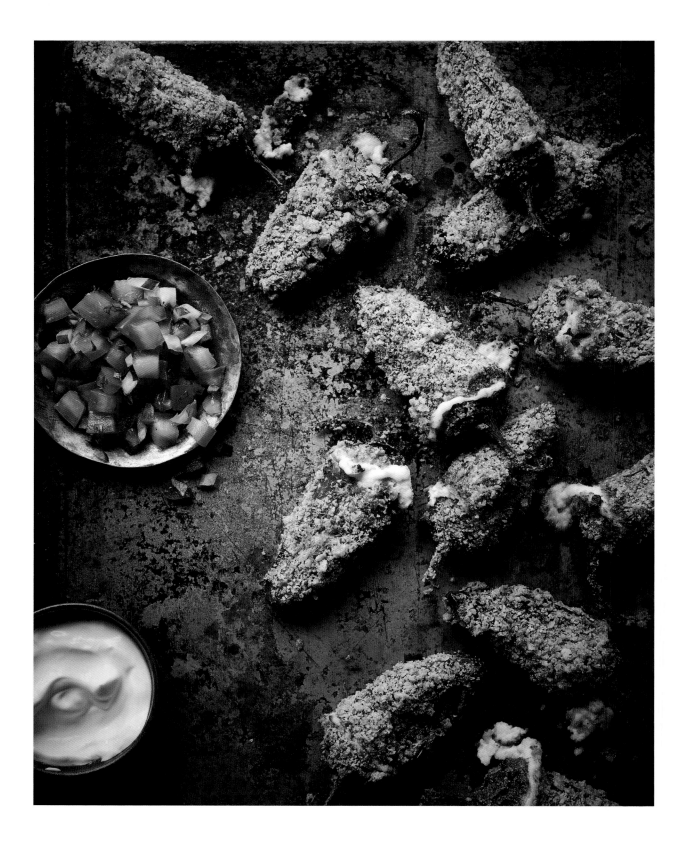

Jalapeño Poppers

... *for the Brave*

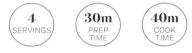

These tasty, crunchy (and super spicy) jalapeño poppers ooze a creamy Cheddar filling. They are coated in my keto-friendly crumb before being baked to perfection. The macros are based on this serving four brave souls as part of a tapas spread and exclude any garnishes. However, as I'm sure you already know, when it comes to jalapeño poppers, soured cream and fresh tomato salsa (see page 32) are a must!

CALORIES 179 | CARBOHYDRATES 4.5G | PROTEIN 11G | FAT 12G

4 SERVINGS

30m PREP TIME

40m COOK TIME

200g (7oz) fresh jalapeños

100g (3½oz) full-fat cream cheese

25g (1oz) extra-mature full-fat Cheddar cheese, finely grated

1 large egg, whisked

salt flakes and salt

For the keto crumb

35g (1¼oz) lean pork scratchings

1 tablespoon nutritional yeast flakes

½ tablespoon almond flour

½ tablespoon finely grated Parmesan cheese

¼ teaspoon garlic powder

generous pinch of salt

To serve

soured cream (optional)

Dynamite Salsa (see page 32) (optional)

Preheat the oven to 200°C/180°C fan/400°F/gas mark 6 and line a large baking tray with baking paper.

Bring a large saucepan of water to the boil. Once it's boiling, add the jalapeños and cook for 5 minutes, then remove using a slotted spoon and plunge into a bowl of iced water. Once cooled, drain well and place the jalapeños on a baking tray lined with paper towels. Gently pat dry, then use a small, sharp knife to carefully make a cut about 1cm (½in) from the stalk end of each jalapeño, cutting only three-quarters of the way through. You want the end to open like a lid, but still be attached.

Gently scrape around inside each jalapeño, loosening the inner parts that contain the seeds. Empty the inside of any excess moisture.

For the filling, simply combine the cream cheese and Cheddar in a little bowl. Season with salt and scoop into a piping bag. Pipe the cream cheese mixture into the hollow jalapeños, filling each one completely. 'Seal' the little stalk lids by gently pressing them down.

For the keto crumb, put the pork scratchings in a mini food processor and blitz to a fine crumb. Tip into a bowl and stir in all the remaining crumb ingredients. Spread out the mixture on a second large tray.

Place the whisked egg in a small bowl and (working one at a time), dip each jalapeño lightly in the whisked egg, allowing any excess to run off, then place on the tray of crumb, leaving a little space in between each one. Gently roll them around until all the jalapeños are evenly coated in the crumb mixture. Carefully transfer the coated jalapeños to the prepared baking tray and bake for 25–30 minutes. They are best eaten hot and crispy with all the lovely trimmings on the side.

Crumbed Mushrooms

2 SERVINGS

20m PREP TIME

30m COOK TIME

These moreish crumbed mushrooms are delicious served with a roast garlic aioli (included in the macros). If you'd like to make one, simply place 5 whole garlic cloves, with their skins still on, on a small sheet of foil. Drizzle over a little olive oil and wrap tightly to make a foil 'parcel', ensuring there are no holes. Roast at 160°C/140°C fan/325°F/ gas mark 3 for 45 minutes. Once cool enough to handle, unwrap the foil and snip off the ends of each clove. Squeeze the roasted flesh into 80g (2¾oz) mayonnaise, and mix well to combine. Simple and delicious!

CALORIES 462 | CARBOHYDRATES 5G | PROTEIN 17G | FAT 41G

Preheat the oven to 200°C/180°C fan/400°F/ gas mark 6 and line a baking tray with baking paper.

1 large egg, whisked

200g (7oz) mushrooms (any larger ones halved)

salt flakes

small handful of fresh flat-leaf parsley, finely chopped, to garnish

For the keto crumb coating

35g (1¼oz) lean pork scratchings

1 tablespoon nutritional yeast flakes

½ tablespoon almond flour

½ tablespoon finely grated Parmesan cheese

¼ teaspoon garlic powder

generous pinch of salt

Put the pork scratchings in a mini food processor and blitz to a fine crumb. Tip into a bowl and stir in the nutritional yeast flakes, almond flour, grated Parmesan, garlic powder and salt. Spread out the crumb on a second large tray.

Place the whisked egg in a bowl and add the mushrooms, tossing to evenly coat. Transfer the mushrooms to a colander, allowing all the excess egg to drain off. Place each mushroom on the tray of crumb, leaving a little space in between each one. This will allow you to gently roll them around until they are evenly coated in the crumb mixture. Transfer the coated mushrooms on to the prepared baking tray and bake for 25–30 minutes.

When the mushrooms are ready and the crumb has crisped up beautifully, season them with salt flakes and scatter over the finely chopped parsley. Serve with the delicious roast garlic aioli (see above).

*

I have tried these in an air fryer, too, and it works great. Keep checking on them, though, as mine took only 15 minutes in the air fryer.

Fried Mozzarella Balls

2 SERVINGS **10m** PREP TIME **5m** COOK TIME

These fried mozzarella balls are coated in my keto batter (a creation I am so, so proud of!) and are delicately crunchy on the outside and gooey on the inside: tapas heaven! Once you have mastered working with the batter, why not try battered onion rings or even battered prawns? For more inspiration, check out my Battered Squid Rings (page 54) and Battered Fish (page 67).

CALORIES 282 | CARBOHYDRATES 6.8G | PROTEIN 13G | FAT 22G

120g (4¼oz) baby mozzarella balls (pearls), drained well

1 large egg white

1 tablespoon double cream

2 tablespoons arrowroot powder (or use 2 x 8g/¼oz sachets)

1 teaspoon baking powder

½ teaspoon paprika

ghee, for deep-frying

1 teaspoon psyllium husk powder

salt flakes, salt and ground white pepper

Place the drained mozzarella balls on a plate lined with paper towels and cover with another layer of paper towels. We need them to be as dry as possible so the batter sticks to them. Set aside.

In a small bowl, whisk together the egg white, cream, arrowroot powder, baking powder and paprika. Season with salt and ground white pepper.

Add enough ghee for deep-frying to a medium-sized saucepan and place over a high heat until it is very hot. Have a plate lined with paper towels at the ready, as well as a slotted spoon or spider strainer.

Once you are ready to deep-fry, whisk the psyllium husk powder into the bowl of batter. If your batter is left to stand for too long, the psyllium husk powder will thicken the mixture far too much, so it's important to do it at the last moment. (If you find it does over-thicken, just whisk in a small dash of cream or egg white to loosen it up again.)

Work in 2–3 batches to avoid overcrowding the pan. Working quickly, add the first batch of mozzarella balls to the batter and stir to evenly coat. Using 2 cocktail sticks, lift each mozzarella ball from the batter and drop it into the hot ghee. Try to avoid letting them touch each other.

They won't take long to cook at all – just a few seconds. If you feel they are turning too golden too quickly for your liking, you can reduce the temperature of the ghee slightly. Use a slotted spoon or spider strainer to remove the coated balls from the pan and place them on the paper-towel-lined plate. Repeat with the remaining balls. Scatter over some salt flakes and serve immediately.

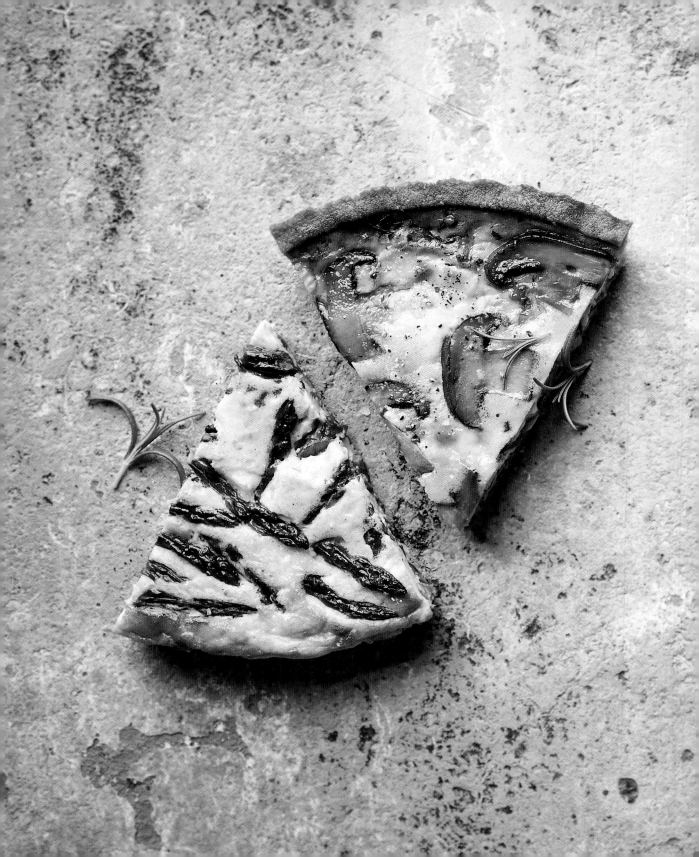

Keto Meals & Side Dish Ideas

Mushroom & Camembert Tart

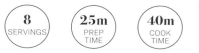

8 SERVINGS **25m** PREP TIME **40m** COOK TIME

I love food that offers massive flavour, and this indulgent mushroom and Camembert tart is a perfect example! While I absolutely love meat and fish, a slice or two of this vegetarian tart makes for a beautiful and filling meal when enjoyed with a fresh, acidic salad on the side. Do not omit the generous amount of finely chopped fresh rosemary needles in the mix: their flavour brings all the elements together beautifully. The macros are calculated per slice, assuming you slice the tart into eight pieces. *Pictured on page 42.*

CALORIES 320 | CARBOHYDRATES 3.9G | PROTEIN 9.9G | FAT 29G

For the crust

140g (5oz) almond flour

1 teaspoon garlic powder

1 large egg white, lightly whisked

40g (1½oz) unsalted butter, melted

pinch of salt

For the filling

2 tablespoons unsalted butter

400g (14oz) mushrooms, sliced or chopped

3 garlic cloves, finely chopped

4–5 rosemary sprigs, needles finely chopped

70g (2½oz) Camembert cheese, broken up into small pieces

2 large eggs

100ml (3½fl oz) double cream

50g (1¾oz) full-fat cream cheese

50g (1¾oz) soured cream

*

If you have some truffle-infused olive oil at hand, a small drizzle over the baked tart will lift the flavour even further!

Preheat the oven to 200°C/180°C fan/400°F/gas mark 6 and line a 22cm (8½in) loose-bottomed fluted tart tin with baking paper.

Begin by making the crust. In a bowl, mix together the almond flour, garlic powder and a pinch of salt. Pour in the lightly whisked egg white and mix well before adding the melted butter (which should not be piping hot, otherwise it will cook parts of the egg). Once combined, tip the mixture into the prepared tin, pressing it along the bottom and up the sides in an even, compact layer. This might be tricky if the mixture is still warm, so leave it for a few minutes to cool so that it won't stick to your fingers. Use a fork to lightly poke a few holes in the base (not all the way through). Bake for 14–15 minutes, then remove from the oven and set aside on a wire rack. Leave the oven on.

Meanwhile, to make the filling, melt the butter in a large non-stick frying pan or wok over a high heat. Once it's foaming, add the mushrooms and cook for 8–10 minutes until they release all their moisture and start to caramelise. Add the garlic and rosemary and reduce the heat to medium. Cook for 3–4 minutes, stirring regularly, until the mixture is free from all moisture and the garlic has softened. Tip into the cooled baked tart case. Scatter the Camembert pieces over the top of the mushroom mixture.

Whisk the eggs, cream, cream cheese and soured cream together in a bowl, ensuring there are no lumps. Pour the mixture into the tart case, over the mushrooms and Camembert.

Bake for 22–23 minutes, rotating halfway through to ensure the tart cooks evenly. Insert a skewer into the centre to check it is cooked: it should come out clean. Remove from the oven and allow to cool a little in the tin before carefully removing and slicing.

Asparagus & Three-cheese Quiche

Deliciously rich and packed with flavour, this crustless quiche is an excellent option for a light lunch. I simply could not have packed more rich cheese into it, even if I wanted to! Slice it as you please, but the macros are calculated assuming you are slicing it into eight pieces. *Pictured on page 42.*

8 SERVINGS | **15m** PREP TIME | **40m** COOK TIME

CALORIES 225 | CARBOHYDRATES 1.9G | PROTEIN 6.5G | FAT 21G

250g (9oz) fine asparagus, trimmed (trimmed weight)

1 tablespoon unsalted butter

3 large eggs

180ml (6fl oz) double cream

75g (2¾oz) full-fat cream cheese

75g (2¾oz) soured cream

2 tablespoons finely grated Parmesan cheese

40g (1½oz) extra-mature full-fat Cheddar cheese, finely grated

salt, salt flakes, ground white pepper and freshly ground black pepper

*

Keeping the asparagus tips separate to garnish the top of the quiche is for aesthetic purposes only, so if you prefer, you can just mix them in.

Preheat the oven to 200°C/180°C fan/400°F/gas mark 6 and line a 22cm (8½in) loose-bottomed tart tin with baking paper.

Chop the trimmed asparagus stalks into very small pieces (about 1cm/½in), keeping the tips a little longer for aesthetic purposes.

Bring a large saucepan of salted water to the boil and cook the asparagus for 2 minutes before draining well in a colander. (If your asparagus stalks are large, they may need a little more time.)

Melt the butter in a frying pan over a medium heat. Add the asparagus and toss it in the butter. Set aside.

In a bowl, whisk together the eggs, cream, cream cheese and soured cream, ensuring there are no lumps. Season with salt and ground white pepper. Stir through the finely grated Parmesan and Cheddar. Separate out the longer asparagus tips and set them aside, then add the smaller pieces of cooked asparagus stalks to the cheese mixture and stir (see Tip).

Pour the mixture into the prepared tart tin and place it on a baking tray. Arrange the asparagus tips on top. Bake for 20 minutes, then turn off the oven and open the oven door slightly. Leave the quiche to finish cooking gently in the residual heat for another 10–15 minutes. When it's ready, the centre should be a little wobbly, but not runny. A cocktail stick inserted in the centre is a useful way to double check: it should come out clean. Allow to cool a little before carefully removing from the tart tin and slicing. Season with salt flakes (if needed) and a crack of freshly ground black pepper.

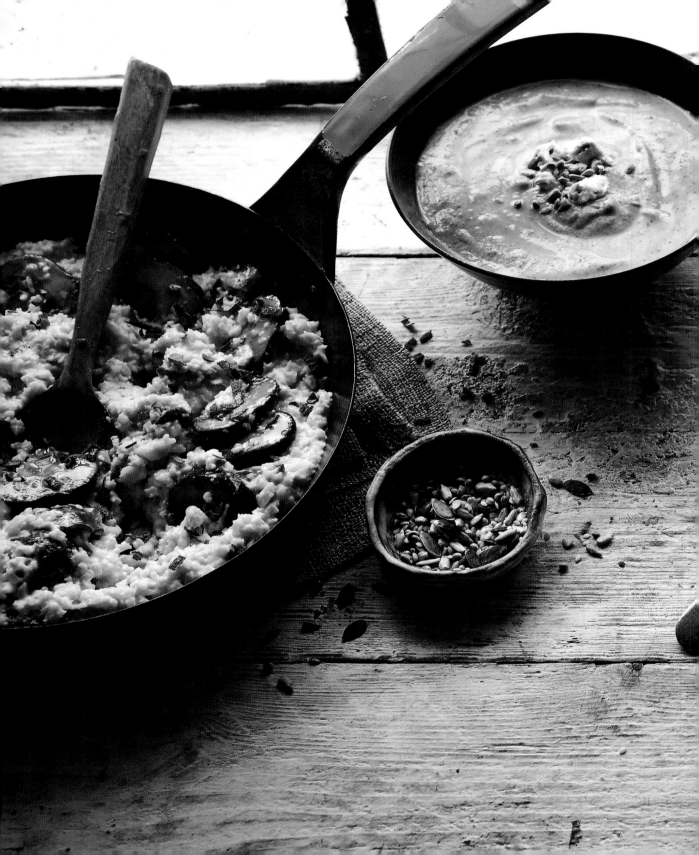

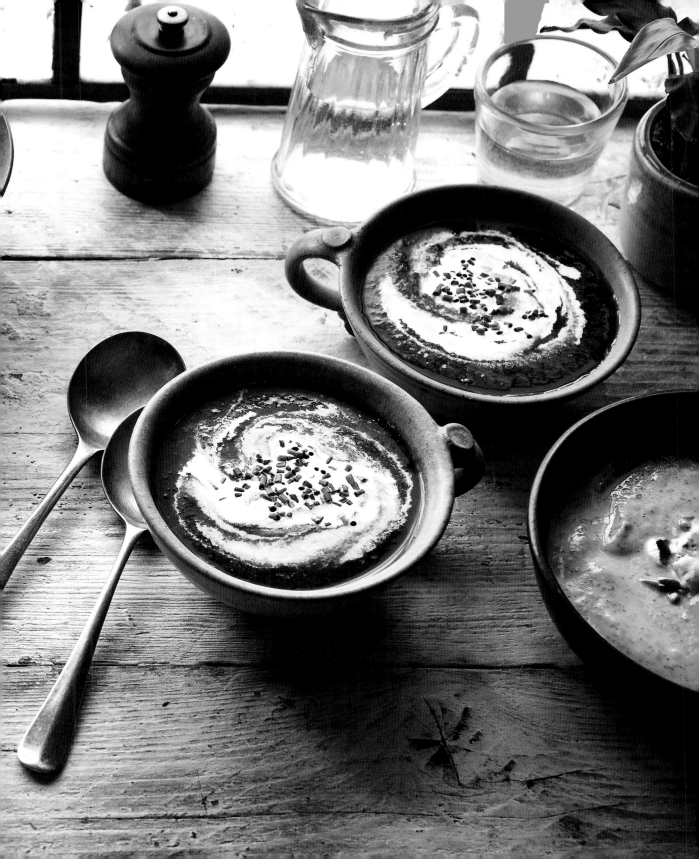

Broccoli & Blue Cheese Soup

Broccoli is one of my favourite vegetables, and the blue cheese adds a sharp flavour that I love. This soup is ideal for the chillier months and can be enjoyed in a cup (making four servings) or in hearty, generous bowlfuls, serving two (as the macros indicate). *Pictured on page 46.*

2 SERVINGS   **5m** PREP TIME   **25m** COOK TIME

CALORIES 434 | CARBOHYDRATES 9.1G | PROTEIN 26G | FAT 31G

1 litre (1¾ pints) best-quality chicken stock

450g (1lb) broccoli florets

50g (1¾oz) soured cream

50g (1¾oz) blue cheese

2 tablespoons double cream

1 teaspoon mixed seeds, to garnish (optional)

Pour the chicken stock into a large, wide saucepan and bring to the boil. Add the broccoli and boil for 10–15 minutes, partly covered, until completely softened

Remove the pan from the heat and use a hand blender, right there in the pan, to blitz the mixture to a smooth consistency. Stir in the soured cream and crumble in most of the blue cheese (setting a little aside to garnish).

Return the pan to the heat and allow the mixture to warm through gently before dividing the soup between 2 warm bowls. Swirl 1 tablespoon of cream into each bowl and top with the remaining blue cheese, along with some mixed seeds (if using).

Cuppa Creamy Tomato Soup

This is my version of my *gunstelling* (favourite) soup as a child in South Africa, and it brings back all the feels. Adding grated Parmesan enriches the flavour further. I advise you enjoy just a cupful as a light meal, because the carbs in tomatoes can add up! *Pictured on page 47.*

4 SERVINGS   **5m** PREP TIME   **25m** COOK TIME

CALORIES 180 | CARBOHYDRATES 7.9G | PROTEIN 4.8G | FAT 14G

2 x 400g (14oz) cans chopped tomatoes

400ml (14fl oz) best-quality chicken stock

2 tablespoons finely grated Parmesan cheese (optional)

100ml (3½fl oz) double cream, plus extra to drizzle

salt and ground white pepper

freshly chopped chives, to garnish (optional)

Pour the canned tomatoes into a large saucepan. Add the chicken stock and bring to the boil. Reduce the heat to low and simmer (partially covered) for 15 minutes, stirring regularly.

Remove from the heat and use a hand blender, right there in the pan, to blitz the mixture to a smooth consistency. If you're using Parmesan, add it halfway through blitzing. Stir in the cream and return the pan to the heat to gently warm the soup through. Season with salt and white pepper and divide between 4 cups. Drizzle with a little extra cream for a pretty presentation, and garnish with chopped chives (if using).

Mushroom & Sage Caulisotto

This cauliflower risotto features fantastic flavours from the caramelised mushrooms and fresh sage, a beautiful herb we often only associate with pork. Remember, if you prefer to keep this dish vegetarian-friendly, use nutritional yeast flakes (see page 9 for more info) in place of Parmesan, as it offers the same punchy, 'cheesy' flavour. *Pictured on page 46.*

2 SERVINGS | **15m** PREP TIME | **25m** COOK TIME

CALORIES 474 | CARBOHYDRATES 9.6G | PROTEIN 14G | FAT 41G

300g (10½oz) cauliflower florets

2 tablespoons unsalted butter

200g (7oz) mushrooms, thickly sliced

2 garlic cloves, finely sliced

50ml (2fl oz) dry white wine

90ml (6 tablespoons) double cream

30g (1oz) Parmesan cheese, finely grated

7–8 fresh sage leaves, thinly sliced

salt flakes, salt, ground white pepper and freshly ground black pepper

squeeze of fresh lemon juice, to serve

Place the cauliflower in a food processor and blitz until it resembles coarse breadcrumbs. (If you are using a mini food processor, this is best done in 2 or 3 batches.) Transfer to a wide, shallow, microwave-safe bowl and microwave on high for 5 minutes, then carefully remove and set aside.

Melt a third of the butter in a large non-stick frying pan or wok over a high heat. Once it's foaming, add half of the mushrooms and fry until they are golden and caramelised on the outside. Remove and set aside on a plate, seasoning with salt and ground white pepper. Repeat the process with another third of the butter and the remaining mushrooms and set aside on the plate, seasoning as before.

Reduce the heat to medium–low and add the remaining butter. Add the garlic and cook until softened, then pour in the white wine. Cook until all the wine has evaporated.

Once there is no more moisture in the pan, add the cooked cauliflower 'rice' and the caramelised mushrooms, along with the double cream, grated Parmesan and most of the sliced sage. Stir to combine and gently warm all the elements through.

Serve immediately, scattered with salt flakes, freshly ground black pepper and the remaining sage, to garnish. A generous squeeze of lemon juice will bring it all together perfectly.

Sea Bass

with Browned Garlic Butter & Herbs

Here, my sea bass is cooked skin-side down to achieve a lovely crispy skin, before being gently finished skin-side up in a warm oven. I then drizzle over a browned garlic butter to maximise flavour, before finishing with a generous combination of herbs. Lush! I recommend you enjoy this with the Broccoli & Asparagus with Lemon Dressing (page 118) as pictured, because it contains tarragon and capers, which complement fish beautifully. This is an easy midweek fish dinner, but I think it could become your latest dinner party dazzler!

4 SERVINGS | 15m PREP TIME | 15m COOK TIME

CALORIES 237 | CARBOHYDRATES 0.5G | PROTEIN 19G | FAT 18G

4 boneless sea bass fillets (approx. 95g/3¼oz per fillet), skin on

3 tablespoons unsalted butter

2 garlic cloves, very finely sliced (see Tip)

1 teaspoon finely chopped fresh oregano leaves

1 teaspoon finely chopped fresh mint leaves

1 teaspoon finely chopped fresh flat-leaf parsley leaves

salt flakes, salt and ground white pepper

lemon wedges, to serve

*

The garlic should be very finely sliced, as it will not be on the heat for long. If you accidentally burn the garlic, simply strain the butter to remove it before pouring it over the fish.

Preheat the oven to 120°C/100°C fan/250°F/gas mark ½ and line a baking tray with baking paper.

Remove the fish from its packaging and pat dry with paper towels – particularly the skin side. Season all sides with salt and ground white pepper. Melt 1 tablespoon of the butter in a large non-stick frying pan over a high heat and cook the fish, skin-side down, for 2–3 minutes until golden and crispy. (Sea bass tends to curl as soon as it hits a hot pan, so use your spatula to flatten the fillets down to ensure even crisping of the skin.)

Remove the fish fillets from the pan and place them, skin-side up, on the prepared baking tray. Transfer to the oven for 9–10 minutes to gently finish cooking while you make the brown garlic butter.

Heat the remaining 2 tablespoons of butter in a small, clean saucepan over a medium heat until it starts to foam. You will soon notice a lovely nutty aroma as the butter stops foaming and the milk solids start to brown. When you notice this, immediately remove the pan from the heat and add the finely sliced garlic, which will gently cook in the hot butter and take on some colour.

Pour the browned butter and garlic over the cooked fish, and scatter generously with the finely chopped herbs. Season with salt flakes and serve with lemon wedges alongside.

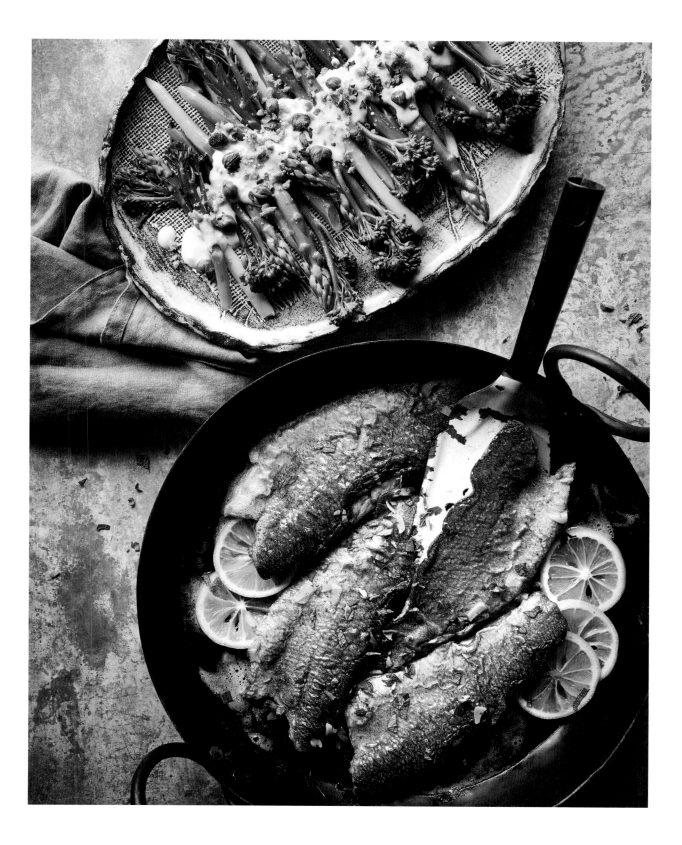

Spicy Moroccan Seafood

This fantastically spicy seafood dish reminds me of one I had in Essaouira, Morocco a few years back. It's great to serve for guests as it can be prepared the day before and reheated (see Tip). I used frozen mussels in this recipe because my local supermarket sells the frozen cooked meat (without shell). If you like, you can also opt for frozen fish and seafood (which is often more affordable) – just defrost it before using by laying it out on a tray lined with paper towels and leaving it in the refrigerator overnight.

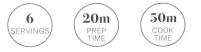

6 SERVINGS   **20m** PREP TIME   **50m** COOK TIME

CALORIES 209 | CARBOHYDRATES 9G | PROTEIN 29G | FAT 6.1G

1 tablespoon unsalted butter

½ onion, finely chopped

3 garlic cloves, finely chopped

25g (1oz) red chilli, finely chopped

2 tablespoons harissa paste

1 teaspoon smoked paprika

1 teaspoon ground cumin

1 teaspoon ground ginger

400g (14oz) chopped tomatoes, canned or fresh

1 tablespoon double-concentrate tomato purée

400ml (14fl oz) best-quality fish stock

1 cinnamon stick

250g (9oz) skinless uncooked white fish fillets, cut into chunks

250g (9oz) uncooked squid tubes, cut into rings

250g (9oz) uncooked king prawns, peeled

200g (7oz) cooked mussels, defrosted if using frozen

80g (2¾oz) full-fat plain yogurt

zest and juice of 1 lemon

salt and freshly ground black pepper

small handful of fresh flat-leaf parsley leaves, finely chopped, to garnish

Melt the butter in a large non-stick frying pan or wok over a medium heat. Add the onion and cook for 10–12 minutes until softened. Add the garlic, chilli, harissa paste, smoked paprika, cumin and ginger, and continue to cook for 1–2 minutes until the pan looks dry.

Tip in the chopped tomatoes, tomato purée, fish stock and cinnamon stick. Bring to the boil, then reduce the heat to low and simmer, uncovered, for 25 minutes until the mixture thickens, stirring occasionally.

Add all the fish and seafood and allow to gently poach in the hot mixture for 10–12 minutes.

Pick out and discard the cinnamon stick and season the mixture with salt and freshly ground black pepper. Stir through the yogurt and finish with a generous scattering of lemon zest and parsley. A good squeeze of lemon juice (catch the pips!) will finish the dish beautifully. Serve over seasoned cauliflower rice, courgette noodles or any of your favourite konjac (shirataki) products (excluded in these macros).

*

If you make this ahead of time, gently reheat over a medium heat for 10–15 minutes, adding the yogurt, lemon and herb garnishes just before serving.

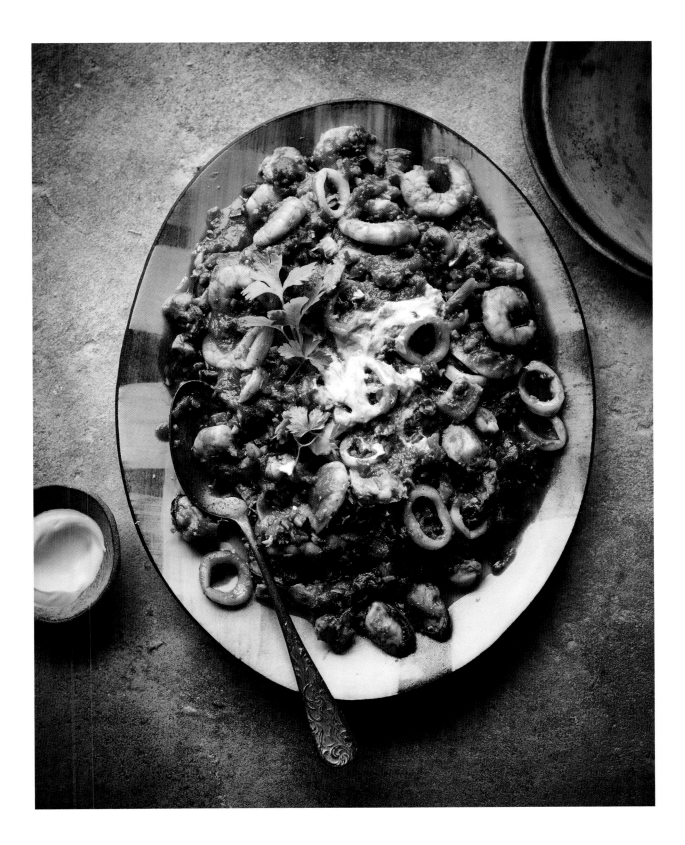

Fried calamari was always my first choice if it featured on a menu when eating out, but once I started eating keto, it was no longer an option... until now! I am pleased to say that I can still enjoy it at home after developing my keto batter. These squid rings would be delicious with the Tartare Sauce featured on page 67. If 8.6g carbs seems a little hefty, share this platter between four people as an appetiser instead.

CALORIES 238 | CARBOHYDRATES 8.6G | PROTEIN 21G | FAT 13G

Battered Squid Rings

2 SERVINGS

10m PREP TIME

20m COOK TIME

1 large egg white

1 tablespoon double cream

2 tablespoons arrowroot powder (or use 2 x 8g/¼oz sachets)

1 teaspoon baking powder

½ teaspoon paprika

ghee, for deep-frying

½ teaspoon psyllium husk powder

250g (9oz) uncooked squid rings, drained well and patted dry with paper towels

salt flakes, salt and ground white pepper

freshly chopped flat-leaf parsley and lemon wedges, to serve

In a small bowl, whisk together the egg white, cream, arrowroot powder, baking powder and paprika. Season with salt and ground white pepper.

Add enough ghee for deep-frying to a medium-sized saucepan and place over a high heat until it is very hot. Have a plate lined with paper towels at the ready, as well as a slotted spoon or spider strainer.

Once you are ready to deep-fry, whisk the psyllium husk powder into the bowl of batter. If your batter is left to stand for too long, the psyllium husk powder will thicken the mixture far too much, so it's important to do it at the last moment. (If you find it does over-thicken, just whisk in a small dash of cream or egg white to loosen it up again.)

Working quickly, add all the squid rings to the batter and gently combine to evenly coat. I thread the coated squid rings on to a chopstick to allow me to drop them into the hot ghee a few at a time. In order to avoid the pieces touching each other, it is best to fry them in batches.

Deep-fry the rings until golden brown – this won't take long (less than a minute) – then use a slotted spoon or spider strainer to remove them from the pan and transfer them to the paper towel-lined plate. Scatter over some salt flakes and the chopped parsley and serve immediately to ensure the batter remains crispy, with some lemon wedges ready for squeezing.

Fishcakes
with Tamari Mayo

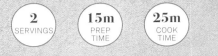

These fishcakes are so easy to make, but work carefully with them: they're delicate in flavour, but they're delicate in texture, too. The tamari mayo is simply heavenly. If you prefer not to use tamari, coconut aminos is an excellent alternative.

CALORIES 316 | CARBOHYDRATES 0.6G | PROTEIN 29G | FAT 21G

100ml (3½fl oz) double cream

150ml (5fl oz) water

1 dried bay leaf

1 teaspoon whole black peppercorns

300g (10½oz) skinless, boneless cod fillets (or any other white fish), patted dry with paper towels

2 spring onions, finely sliced

finely grated zest of 1 lemon

1 large egg white

1 teaspoon psyllium husk powder

2 teaspoons ghee

salt and ground white pepper

For the tamari mayo

30g (1oz) mayonnaise

1½ teaspoons tamari (gluten-free soy sauce)

Place the cream, water, bay leaf and peppercorns in a medium-sized saucepan and bring to the boil. As soon as the mixture starts to boil, turn off the heat and immediately lower the cod fillets into the pan until completely submerged. Leave to gently poach for 10 minutes.

Drain the fish well, discarding the poaching liquid. Be sure to pick out any hidden peppercorns. Place the fish in a bowl and allow to cool a little before using a fork to thoroughly flake the flesh. Add the sliced spring onions (setting aside a few of the green ends to use later as a garnish), along with the lemon zest, egg white and psyllium husk powder. Season generously with salt and white pepper and mix well. Leave to sit for a minute to allow the psyllium husk powder to thicken the mixture, making it more workable. Form the mixture into 6 evenly sized fishcakes (approximately 55g/2oz each). If you aren't cooking them straight away, keep covered in the refrigerator until needed.

Preheat the oven to 120°C/100°C fan/250°F/gas mark ½.

To cook the fishcakes, I advise you work in 2 batches. Heat 1 teaspoon of the ghee in a large non-stick frying pan over a high heat. Add the first 3 fishcakes and cook for 1–2 minutes until golden. Turn them gently and reduce the heat to medium. Cover the pan with a lid or foil and cook for an additional 5 minutes to ensure the egg white is cooked through. Remove from the heat. Place in the warm oven while you repeat the process with the remaining ghee and fishcakes.

For the tamari mayo, simply whisk together the mayonnaise and tamari in a small bowl. Serve the warm fishcakes with the tamari mayo drizzled over, garnished with the greens ends of the spring onions.

Salmon & Avocado Poke Bowl

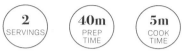

(**2** SERVINGS) (**40m** PREP TIME) (**5m** COOK TIME)

Sushi-grade salmon would be ideal for this recipe, but in all honesty, I do not generally bother sourcing it: I simply use the freshest salmon I can find, because the fish gets 'cooked' in the acidic lime juice in much the same way as a ceviche. The lovely, fresh flavours in this bowl are unbeatable. My husband loves it with just a bit of heat, so he sprinkles over a pinch of dried chilli flakes. It is fresh and filling, and perfect for summer!

CALORIES 553 | CARBOHYDRATES 5.7G | PROTEIN 36G | FAT 41G

260g (9¼oz) skinless salmon fillets (see Tip), cut into small, bite-sized pieces

juice of 1 lime

1 tablespoon tamari (gluten-free soy sauce)

200g (7oz) cauliflower florets

2 teaspoons rice wine vinegar

4 spring onions, finely sliced

2 teaspoons toasted sesame oil

1 avocado, peeled, stoned and sliced

1 teaspoon sesame seeds

squeeze of fresh lime juice (optional)

small handful of fresh coriander leaves, finely chopped, to garnish

dried chilli flakes, to garnish (optional)

*

If you cannot source skinless salmon, remove the skin from the fillets using a small, sharp knife. Do not discard the skins – fry them in a little butter until golden and crispy for a delicious treat!

Place the salmon in a bowl. Pour over the lime juice and tamari and toss well to evenly coat. Cover and place in the refrigerator for at least 25 minutes while you prepare the remaining ingredients.

Place the cauliflower in a food processor and blitz until it resembles coarse breadcrumbs. (If you are using a mini food processor, this is best done in 2 or 3 batches.) Place the blitzed cauliflower 'rice' into a wide, shallow, microwave-safe bowl and microwave on high for 5 minutes. Set aside to cool, preferably in the refrigerator, for at least 10 minutes. Once cooled, stir through the rice wine vinegar, sliced spring onions and sesame oil.

Arrange the 'rice', salmon and avocado in 2 serving bowls, being sure to drizzle over all the marinade juice from the salmon. Taste for seasoning and texture. If you find it a bit dry, or think it requires additional seasoning, add a little more tamari and sesame oil. If you feel it needs more acidity, a squeeze of fresh lime juice will help. Finish with a pretty scattering of sesame seeds, fresh coriander and dried chilli flakes (if using).

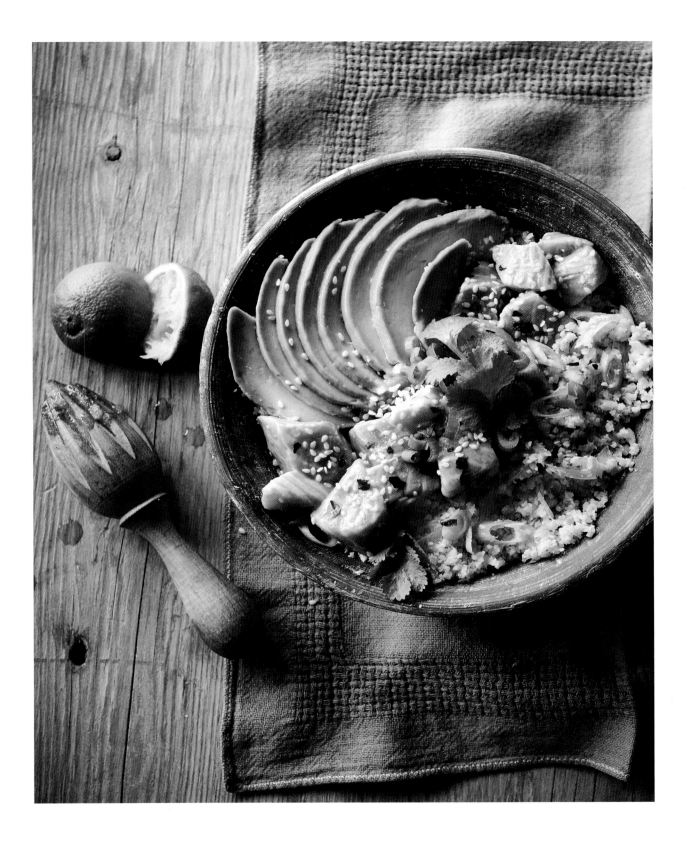

Creamy Lemon Prawn 'Pasta'

This is a deliciously zingy meal packed with massive flavours! I simply flash-fry the prawns, then set them aside while I whip up a quick, creamy sauce. If you choose not to use konjac (shirataki) noodles, this would be equally lovely over courgetti, although the carb count may increase slightly if you choose to do that. *Pictured on page 60.*

2 SERVINGS   **15m** PREP TIME   **10m** COOK TIME

CALORIES 560 | CARBOHYDRATES 4.1G | PROTEIN 24G | FAT 47G

400g (14oz) konjac (shirataki) 'pasta', fettuccine-style

240g (8½oz) peeled raw king prawns

2 tablespoons unsalted butter

2 garlic cloves, finely chopped

juice of 2 lemons

100g (3½oz) soured cream

100ml (3½fl oz) double cream

salt flakes, salt and ground white pepper

small handful of fresh flat-leaf parsley leaves, finely chopped, to garnish

Prepare the konjac 'pasta' according to the instructions on page 7.

Meanwhile, remove the prawns from their packaging and pat dry with paper towels. We are flash-frying them, so any excess moisture present will prevent caramelisation.

It is best to cook the prawns in 2 batches to avoid crowding the pan. Melt the butter in a large frying pan or wok over a high heat. Once foaming, add the first batch of prawns and cook for 1–2 minutes, turning to cook all sides, until they turn pink and partially caramelise. Use tongs or a slotted spoon to remove the prawns from the pan, leaving all the fat in the pan. Set the prawns aside to keep warm and repeat with the second batch, again leaving all the fat in the pan when you remove them.

Reduce the heat to low and add the chopped garlic to the pan. If the pan is too hot, your garlic will instantly burn, so you may even want to turn off the heat completely so the garlic can soften and cook in the residual heat. Once softened, add all the lemon juice and increase the heat to medium, cooking for 2–3 minutes until the lemon juice completely evaporates and you are left with a darker, jammy mixture. Add the soured cream and double cream and season with salt and ground white pepper. Gently warm the sauce through and allow it to thicken a little (a thicker sauce will coat the 'pasta' better).

Drain the prepared 'pasta' well and add it to the pan of creamy sauce. Return the prawns to the pan, and stir well to combine and warm everything through.

Divide between 2 warm bowls and season with salt flakes. Garnish with chopped parsley for a lovely fresh finish.

Cheesy Spicy Tuna Slices

I made this dish one night when I felt like we just needed something different. We regularly eat a well-balanced amount of red meat and oily fish, but there were some challenging times over the 2020 lockdown where I had to raid my pantry and get creative! With this recipe, I took simple canned tuna up a notch and created a mouth-watering meal for four! This simple meal boasts massive flavours and is easy on the wallet, too. *Pictured on page 61.*

4 SERVINGS | **15m** PREP TIME | **55m** COOK TIME

CALORIES 765 | CARBOHYDRATES 5.4G | PROTEIN 32G | FAT 67G

For the crust

45g (1½oz) unsalted butter

120g (4¼oz) almond flour

1 teaspoon paprika

1 large egg, separated

salt

For the filling

220g (7¾oz) canned tuna, drained (drained weight)

2 large eggs

2 teaspoons medium curry powder

1 teaspoon onion powder

1 teaspoon garlic powder

¼ teaspoon cayenne pepper

80g (2¾oz) extra-mature full-fat Cheddar cheese, grated

200ml (7fl oz) double cream

salt and freshly ground black pepper

To finish

80g (2¾oz) soured cream

small handful of fresh flat-leaf parsley leaves, finely chopped, to garnish

Preheat the oven to 200°C/180°C fan/400°F/gas mark 6 and line the base of a 16 x 16cm (6¼ x 6¼in) deep-sided baking dish with baking paper.

Begin by making the crust. Melt the butter in a small saucepan over a low heat, then set aside to cool a little. In a bowl, combine the almond flour, paprika and a generous pinch of salt. Add the egg yolk from the separated egg (setting aside the white for use in the filling). Stir to combine, then pour in the melted butter and mix well.

Tip the mixture into the prepared baking dish, pressing it down to form an even, compact layer on the base. Pierce with a fork a few times and bake for 16–18 minutes. Remove from the oven and set aside while you prepare the filling, but do not turn the oven off.

Place the drained tuna in a large bowl and add the 2 eggs, along with the reserved egg white. Stir in the curry powder, onion powder, garlic powder and cayenne pepper. Add the Cheddar and season the mixture generously with salt and freshly ground black pepper. Mix well to combine.

In a separate bowl, use a hand mixer to whip the double cream to semi-soft peaks. Fold the whipped cream into the tuna mixture, then pour the whole lot into the baking dish over the cooked base.

Bake for 15 minutes, then reduce the temperature to 180°C/160°C fan/350°F/gas mark 4 and bake for an additional 15–20 minutes, or until a skewer inserted into the centre comes out clean.

Remove from the oven and allow to cool slightly before slicing into 4 slices. This is absolutely delicious served with a spoonful of soured cream on top of each slice and a scattering of chopped parsley.

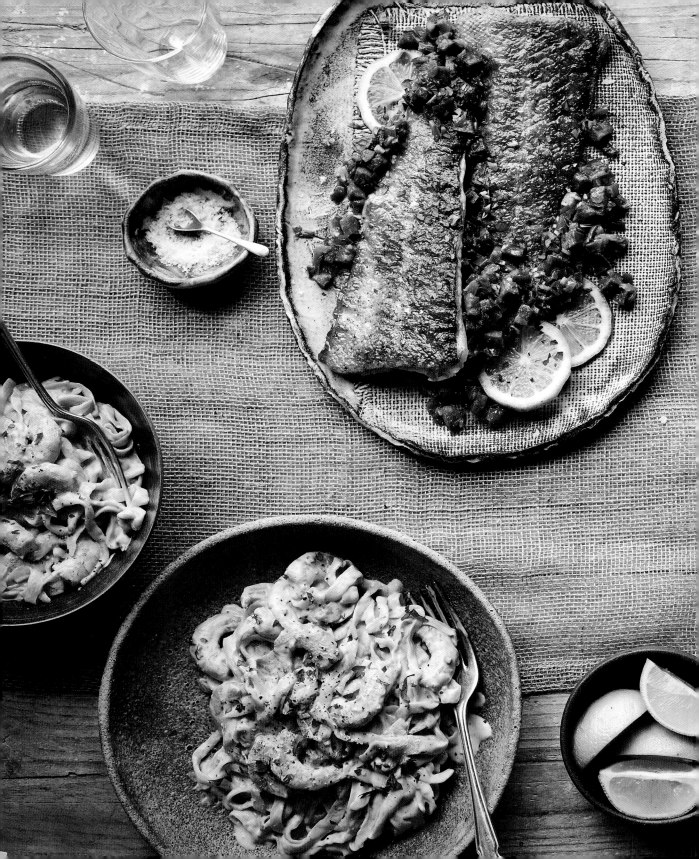

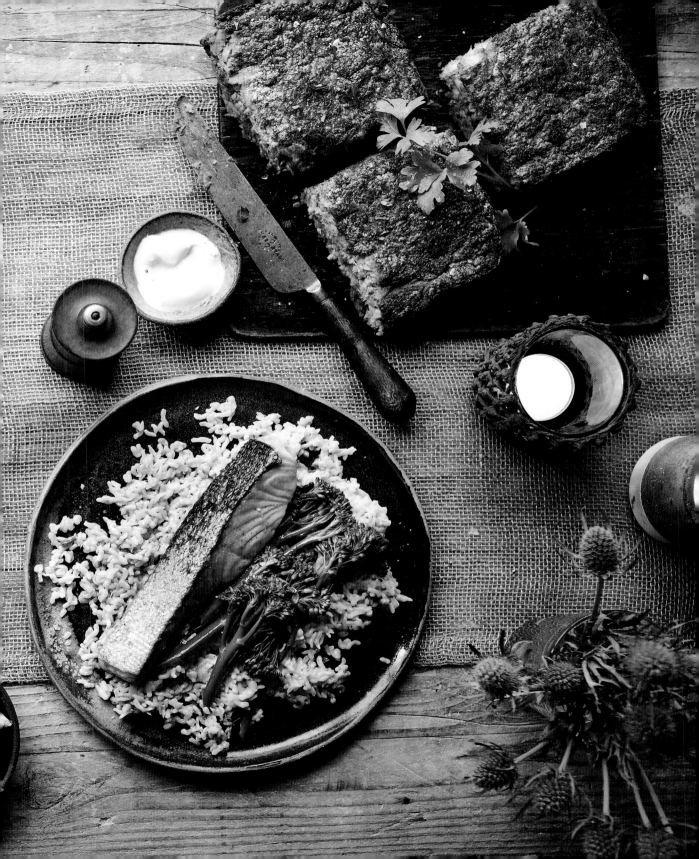

Salmon

with Greens & Ginger Chilli 'Rice'

You are just 30 minutes away from a satisfying, full-flavoured midweek meal that features delicious salmon and a ginger chilli 'rice'. If you choose not to use konjac (shirataki) 'rice' as I suggest, try it with cauliflower rice instead, but I do want to encourage you to give konjac a try. *Pictured on page 61.*

2 SERVINGS | **15m** PREP TIME | **15m** COOK TIME

CALORIES 520 | CARBOHYDRATES 6.3G | PROTEIN 40G | FAT 35G

400g (14oz) konjac (shirataki) 'rice'

200g (7oz) long-stem broccoli, trimmed (trimmed weight)

1 tablespoon unsalted butter

2 salmon fillets, approx. 130g (4¾oz) each, skin-on

2 garlic cloves, finely chopped

25g (1oz) fresh root ginger, peeled and finely minced

1 large red chilli, finely chopped

50g (1¾oz) full-fat cream cheese

1 tablespoon tamari (gluten-free soy sauce)

1 tablespoon toasted sesame oil

salt

Prepare the konjac 'rice' according to the instructions on page 7.

Meanwhile, preheat the oven to 120°C/100°C/250°F/gas mark ½.

Bring a large saucepan of salted water to the boil. Add the broccoli and boil for 4 minutes before draining well. Transfer to an ovenproof dish and cover with foil. Place in the warm oven while you finish the rest of the dish.

Melt the butter in a large non-stick frying pan over a high heat. Once foaming, fry the salmon fillets, skin-side down, for 1 minute until the skins are crispy. Turn them over and cook on the other sides for 3–4 minutes or until done to your liking. Remove from the pan and place in the warm oven with the broccoli.

Using the same frying pan (which still contains all that lovely browned butter), reduce the heat to low and add the garlic, ginger and chilli. Cook for 1–2 minutes until softened. Garlic burns quickly, so stir regularly.

Drain the prepared konjac 'rice' well and tip it into the pan. Add the cream cheese and tamari and stir well to combine, then warm the whole lot through.

Serve the broccoli and salmon on top of the ginger chilli 'rice', and drizzle over the sesame oil to finish.

Cod
with Chorizo & Caramelised Veg

The flavour that a good-quality chorizo brings to a dish is unbeatable. Here, caramelised green peppers and onions are combined with garlic and chopped chorizo and simply served with beautifully cooked cod fillets. Use any white fish you fancy, but be sure it still has the skin on so you can crisp it up for more texture in your dish. Season generously before serving, and don't forget that all-important *squeeeeze* of lemon juice to finish. *Pictured on page 60.*

2 SERVINGS

20m PREP TIME

30m COOK TIME

CALORIES 377 | CARBOHYDRATES 4.7G | PROTEIN 34G | FAT 24G

2 tablespoons unsalted butter

1 green pepper, finely chopped

½ onion, finely chopped

2 garlic cloves, finely chopped

65g (2¼oz) best-quality chorizo, diced small

2 cod fillets (approx. 140g/5oz each), skin on

salt flakes, salt, ground white pepper and freshly ground black pepper

small handful of fresh flat-leaf parsley leaves, finely chopped, to garnish

lemon wedges, to serve

Preheat the oven to 180°C/160°C fan/350°F/gas mark 4.

Melt 1 tablespoon of the butter in a non-stick frying pan or wok over a medium–low heat. Add the green pepper and onion and gently cook until they completely break down and start to caramelise. This can take up to 15 minutes. Add the garlic and chorizo to the pan and cook for a further 2 minutes, stirring regularly to soften the garlic. Set aside to keep warm while you cook the cod.

Remove the fillets from their packaging and pat them dry with paper towels, paying particular attention to the skin side. Season on all sides with salt and ground white pepper. Melt the remaining butter in another large non-stick frying pan over a high heat. Once the butter is sizzling, add the cod fillets, skin-side down. Cook until the skins start to crisp and the butter starts browning. Tilt the pan and use a spoon to scoop up some of the browned butter to drizzle over the flesh side.

Gently lift the cod out of the pan and place, skin-side up, on a baking tray. Place in the oven for no longer than 6–7 minutes to finish cooking through.

Meanwhile, pour the browned butter from frying the fish into the pan of caramelised veg and chorizo, stirring well to combine.

Serve the fish with the caramelised veg, seasoning everything with freshly ground black pepper and salt flakes (if needed). Garnish your masterpiece with chopped parsley, and serve with lemon wedges on the side: a generous squeeze of fresh lemon will finish this dish perfectly.

Monnie's Fish Dugléré

I want to single out this fish dish for a special mention, as it's one of my favourites. It's a beautiful, beautiful dish. You can serve the saucy fish over cauliflower mash or cauliflower 'rice', or you can flake the cooked fish right there in the sauce and serve the whole lot with konjac (shirataki) noodles, as I like to do. Spectacular...

4 SERVINGS | **15m** PREP TIME | **35m** COOK TIME

CALORIES 409 | CARBOHYDRATES 4.2G | PROTEIN 25G | FAT 32G

4 skinless cod fillets, approx. 130g (4¾oz) each, patted dry with paper towels

2 large tomatoes

180ml (6fl oz) double cream

50g (1¾oz) full-fat cream cheese

50g (1¾oz) soured cream

1 tablespoon double-concentrate tomato purée

1 teaspoon unsalted butter

2 garlic cloves, finely chopped

½ lemon

salt flakes, salt and ground white pepper

2–3 fresh thyme sprigs, leaves picked

*

You can use any white fish you like, but it must be boneless and skinless for this recipe. I often use cod loins, which are more generous in size!

Preheat the oven to 200°C/180°C fan/400°F/gas mark 6.

Season the cod with salt and white pepper and place in an ovenproof dish – you want all 4 fillets to fit snugly together in a single layer.

Cut the tomatoes into thin wedges: you want approximately 18–22 little wedges. Use a knife to slide out the fleshy seed area of each wedge. Roughly chop these juicy, seedy bits and set aside for now. Place the deseeded wedges in the dish around the cod fillets.

In a bowl, whisk together the double cream, cream cheese, soured cream and tomato purée until a smooth mixture forms with no lumps.

Melt the butter in a large non-stick frying pan over a low–medium heat. Add the garlic and gently cook for 1–2 minutes until it softens. Stir in the reserved tomato flesh and seeds and squeeze in the juice from the lemon half. Add the squeezed lemon to the pan for an extra zingy flavour. Increase the heat to medium and cook for 5–6 minutes until all the moisture evaporates and you are left with a thick, chunky mixture.

Pour the cream mixture into the pan and increase the heat to high, cooking for 2–3 minutes as the sauce warms through and reduces a little. At this point, you can remove and discard the lemon half. Season with salt and ground white pepper, then pour the sauce into the ovenproof dish, over the cod and tomato wedges.

Bake for 22–25 minutes, rotating halfway through, until the cod is cooked through. Season with salt flakes and freshly picked thyme leaves, and serve over cauliflower mash or cauliflower 'rice' to mop up that lovely sauce. Alternatively, flake the fish in the sauce and serve over konjac (shirataki) noodles for a delicious low-carb meal!

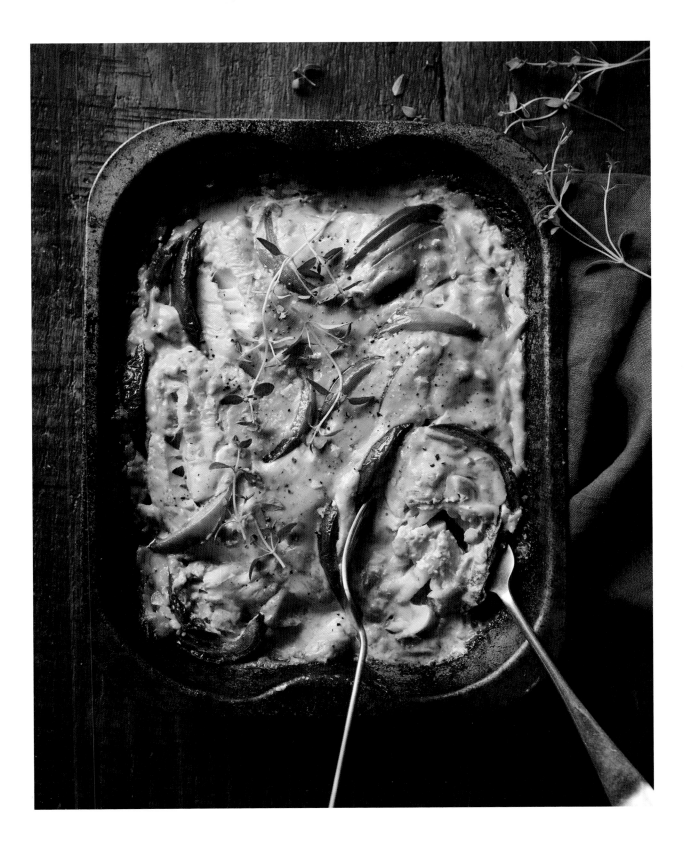

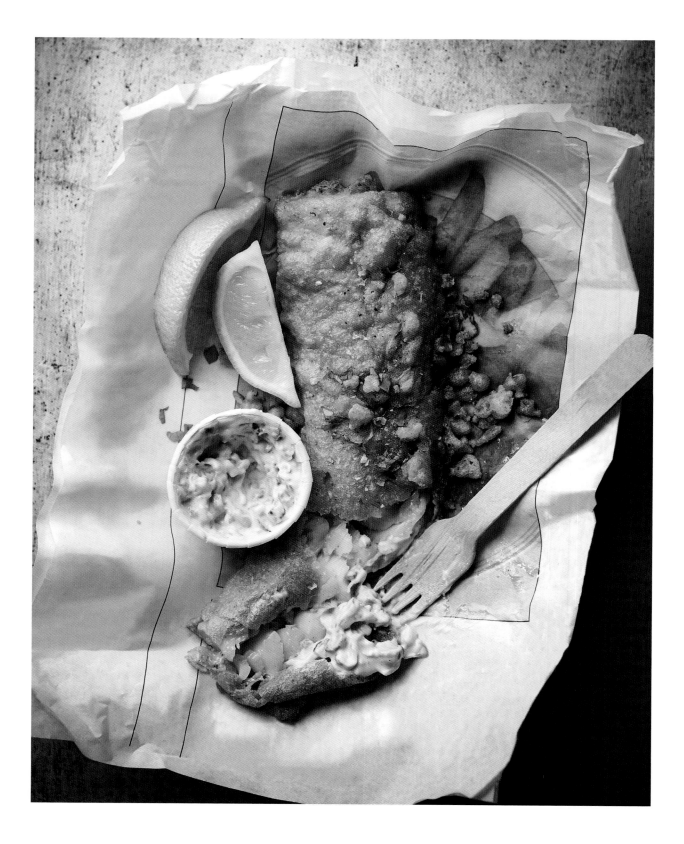

Battered Fish

with Tartare Sauce

I sorely missed my local pub's battered fish after going keto! Can you imagine my delight when these beauties came out so fabulous? My keto batter is delicately crispy and so light: I just know you will love it as much as I do. I have provided a quick and easy tartare sauce which can be enjoyed alongside, and I promise you won't even miss the chips!

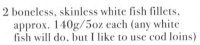

2 SERVINGS | **20m** PREP TIME | **10m** COOK TIME

CALORIES 543 | CARBOHYDRATES 8.7G | PROTEIN 27G | FAT 44G

2 boneless, skinless white fish fillets, approx. 140g/5oz each (any white fish will do, but I like to use cod loins)

1 large egg white

1 tablespoon double cream

2 tablespoons arrowroot powder (or use 2 x 8g/¼oz sachets)

1 teaspoon baking powder

½ teaspoon paprika

ghee, for deep-frying

1 teaspoon psyllium husk powder

salt flakes, salt and ground white pepper

small handful of fresh flat-leaf parsley leaves, finely chopped, to garnish

lemon wedges, to serve

For the tartare sauce

70g (2½oz) mayonnaise

15g (½oz) small capers, finely chopped

15g (½oz) gherkins or cornichons, finely chopped

squeeze of fresh lemon juice

1 tablespoon finely chopped fresh flat-leaf parsley leaves

Begin by making the tartare sauce. Simply combine all the ingredients in a small bowl and set aside.

Remove the fish fillets from their packaging and pat dry using paper towels. This step is essential to allow the batter to adhere to the fish.

In a small bowl, whisk together the egg white, cream, arrowroot powder, baking powder and paprika, and season.

Add enough ghee for deep-frying to a medium-sized saucepan and place over a high heat until it is very hot. Have a plate lined with paper towels at the ready, as well as a slotted spoon or spider strainer.

Once you are ready to deep-fry, whisk the psyllium husk powder into the bowl of batter. If your batter is left to stand for too long, the psyllium husk powder will thicken the mixture far too much, so it's important to do it at the last moment. (If you find it does over-thicken, just whisk in a small dash of cream or egg white to loosen it up again.)

Working quickly, season the fish on all sides with salt and ground white pepper, then dip the fish into the batter and allow any excess batter to run off. Carefully lower the fish into the ghee. Spoon the hot ghee over the top of the fish as it is deep-frying, then gently flip the fish over. Frying fish like this won't take very long (approximately 2–3 minutes, but thicker pieces may require slightly longer cooking times).

Once the fish is golden on all sides, remove with a slotted spoon and place on the paper towel-lined plate.

Serve immediately to ensure the batter remains crispy, seasoned with salt flakes. Scatter over some chopped parsley and serve with lemon wedges and the tartare sauce.

Chicken

with Tomato & Basil 'Couscous'

For this recipe, I created a tasty 'couscous' by baking blitzed cauliflower until partially caramelised. It's delicious served with chicken and my marinated tomato mixture. The fresh basil adds an essential flavour element to this salad, which can be enjoyed warm or cool. So simple and lovely!

2 SERVINGS | **15m** PREP TIME | **40m** COOK TIME

CALORIES 550 | CARBOHYDRATES 7.2G | PROTEIN 51G | FAT 34G

300g (10½oz) cauliflower florets

3 tablespoons olive oil

¼ teaspoon dried oregano

2 boneless, skinless chicken breasts, approx. 170g (6oz) each

1 tablespoon lard or ghee

80g (2¾oz) cherry tomatoes, halved

1 garlic clove, crushed with a garlic press

60g (2¼oz) full-fat feta cheese

4–5 fresh basil leaves, thinly sliced

salt and freshly ground black pepper

Preheat the oven to 220°C/200°C fan/425°F/gas mark 7 and line a large baking tray with baking paper.

Place the cauliflower in a food processor and blitz until it resembles coarse breadcrumbs. (If you are using a mini food processor, this is best done in 2 or 3 batches.) Place the cauliflower 'rice' in a bowl and add 1 tablespoon of the olive oil. Season with salt and combine well to ensure the cauli is completely coated. Transfer to the prepared baking tray and spread out the mixture evenly.

Bake for 10 minutes, then stir, spread out once more and bake for a further 10–12 minutes. Keep an eye on it – if it looks like the edges are burning or it is caramelising too much, you may need to take it out sooner. Tip the cauliflower 'couscous' into a bowl and stir in the oregano. Set aside, but leave the oven on.

Meanwhile, pat the chicken breasts dry using paper towels and season both sides with salt. Heat your fat of choice in a griddle pan over a high heat and fry the breasts for 2–3 minutes until golden on all sides. This caramelisation of the outside adds massive flavour, but the chicken is far from cooked safely, so transfer it to a baking tray and place in the oven for 14–15 minutes until cooked through. Set aside to rest for 5 minutes before slicing.

While the chicken is resting, place the halved cherry tomatoes in a bowl and stir in the crushed garlic. Crumble in the feta and drizzle over 1 tablespoon of the remaining olive oil. Season with a crack of black pepper and stir through the sliced basil.

Arrange the cauli 'couscous' on plates with the tomato mixture and sliced chicken. Drizzle over the remaining olive oil before serving.

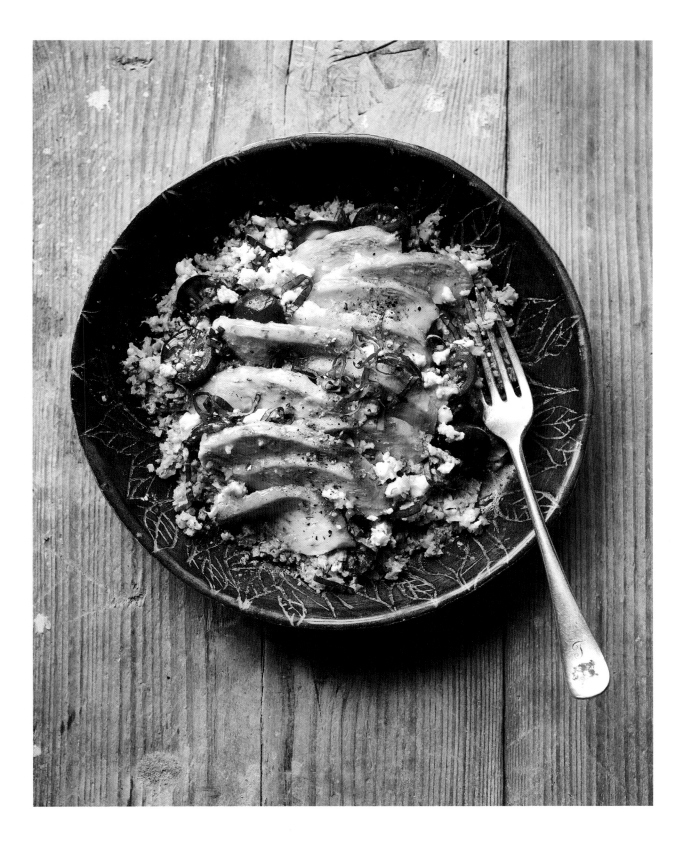

If you like, you can prepare
the chicken 'logs' the day before
and keep them in the refrigerator
overnight before baking the
next day.

Chicken Cordon Bleu

with Creamy Mustard Sauce

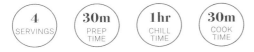

4 SERVINGS | **30m** PREP TIME | **1hr** CHILL TIME | **30m** COOK TIME

This recipe requires a reasonable amount of effort, but the results are superb and will be well worth all the love you put in! A lot of prep can be done ahead of time, but the rich accompanying sauce (which boasts a hint of mustard and nutmeg) should be made just before serving. Serve with simple greens, like steamed broccoli smothered in melted butter. Lush!

CALORIES 916 | CARBOHYDRATES 3.5G | PROTEIN 94G | FAT 58G

4 large boneless, skinless chicken breasts, approx. 230g (8¼oz) each

½ teaspoon garlic powder

8 slices of deli ham, approx. 180g (6½oz) total

8 slices of Emmental cheese, approx. 200g (7oz) total

1 large egg, whisked

salt and ground white pepper

For the keto crumb

70g (2½oz) lean pork scratchings

2 tablespoons nutritional yeast flakes

1 tablespoon almond flour

1 tablespoon finely grated Parmesan cheese

½ teaspoon garlic powder

generous pinch of salt

For the creamy mustard sauce

1 tablespoon unsalted butter

2 garlic cloves, finely chopped

200ml (7fl oz) double cream

40g (1½oz) soured cream

2 tablespoons finely grated Parmesan cheese

2 teaspoons Dijon mustard

pinch of ground nutmeg

Place one of the chicken breasts smooth-side up on a silicone mat. Cover with a large sheet of baking paper and use the flat side of a meat mallet to pound to an even thickness of no more than 1cm (½in), working from the centre of the breast outwards. Remove the top layer of baking paper and gently turn the flattened breast over. Season with salt, ground white pepper and a pinch of garlic powder. Place 2 ham slices on top of the flattened breast and cover with 2 cheese slices. Tuck in the sides, then roll the chicken into a tight 'log'. Wrap in clingfilm, twisting the ends. Repeat with the remaining chicken, seasoning, ham and cheese. Chill for at least 1 hour (see Tip).

Preheat the oven to 200°C/180°C fan/400°F/gas mark 6 and line a baking tray with baking paper.

For the crumb, place the pork scratchings in a mini food processor and blitz well. Stir in the remaining crumb ingredients, then spread out on a second large baking tray. Place the whisked egg in a bowl.

Carefully remove the clingfilm from the chicken and gently roll each 'log' in the whisked egg, lifting it to allow excess egg to run off. Next, roll in the crumb mixture, very gently pressing the crumb into the chicken. Transfer the crumbed chicken 'logs' on to the prepared baking tray and bake for 25–30 minutes. Remove from the oven and allow to rest for at least 5 minutes before slicing.

Meanwhile, make the sauce. Melt the butter in a non-stick saucepan over a low heat and add the garlic. Gently cook for 1–2 minutes until softened, then add all the remaining ingredients. Stir continuously until the mixture is warmed through and has thickened.

Slice and serve the chicken with the sauce and your favourite greens.

A Pot of Chicken Chilli

This easy, delicious one-pan chicken chilli is a variation of the usual beefy chilli con carne. I use chicken thighs here, as they are more succulent than breasts and won't become tough and dry as they simmer. If you are cooking for the kids, adjust the amount of chilli and cayenne pepper, and be sure to serve this with your favourite keto noodles, cauliflower mash or konjac (shirataki) 'rice'. *Pictured on page 75.*

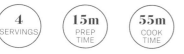

4 SERVINGS | **15m** PREP TIME | **55m** COOK TIME

CALORIES 448 | CARBOHYDRATES 5.3G | PROTEIN 40G | FAT 29G

700g (1lb 9oz) boneless, skinless chicken thighs, cut into bite-sized chunks

2 tablespoons ghee or lard

½ onion, finely chopped

3 garlic cloves, finely chopped

1 red chilli, finely chopped

1½ tablespoons ground cumin

2 teaspoons cayenne pepper

2 teaspoons ground coriander

60ml (4 tablespoons) dry white wine

400ml (14fl oz) best-quality chicken stock

1 tablespoon arrowroot powder

salt and freshly ground black pepper

To serve

70g (2½oz) soured cream

1 red chilli, finely sliced

60g (2¼oz) extra-mature full-fat Cheddar cheese, grated

small handful of fresh coriander leaves, finely chopped

Season the chicken pieces lightly with salt. Heat the ghee or lard in a large, deep-sided non-stick frying pan over a high heat and fry the chicken for 2–3 minutes until golden and crispy on the outside. Remove using tongs and set aside. Do this in 2 or 3 batches so as not to overcrowd the pan, and be mindful that the chicken is still uncooked on the inside, so handle appropriately.

Add the onion to the same pan you used to fry the chicken – it should still contain plenty of fat. Reduce the heat to medium and cook for 5–6 minutes until the onion is softened, then add the garlic and chilli. Cook for a further 1 minute until starting to caramelise. Add the cumin, cayenne pepper and ground coriander and fry lightly for 1 minute more. Deglaze the pan by adding the white wine and cook until all moisture from the wine has evaporated.

Pour a little of the chicken stock into a bowl and add the arrowroot powder. Stir well until dissolved. Pour this mixture into the pan, along with the remaining chicken stock, increasing the heat to bring it to the boil. Stir well to combine.

Once boiling, tip in all the caramelised chicken pieces along with any resting juices, and reduce the heat to low. Simmer for 25–30 minutes until the mixture reduces and completely thickens. By this time, your chicken pieces should have cooked through sufficiently. If in doubt, simply cut open a piece to check.

To finish, stir through the soured cream and season as needed with salt and freshly ground black pepper. Serve garnished with fresh chilli slices, grated Cheddar and plenty of chopped coriander.

Poached Chicken

with Rosemary Butter Sauce

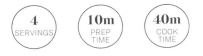

4 SERVINGS | 10m PREP TIME | 40m COOK TIME

I don't often poach chicken breasts, but it's a fantastic technique I wanted to share because it can result in succulent meat if done just right. The poaching liquid then forms the base of a sauce, which is enriched with cream, butter and fresh rosemary. It's unbelievably packed with flavour and may just become your new favourite chicken dinner! *Pictured on page 75.*

CALORIES 421 | CARBOHYDRATES 1.1G | PROTEIN 41G | FAT 27G

4 boneless, skinless chicken breasts, approx. 170g (6oz) each

220ml (7½fl oz) dry white wine

220ml (7½fl oz) water

4 fresh rosemary sprigs, 3 left whole, 1 with needles picked and finely chopped

1 tablespoon whole black peppercorns

3 garlic cloves, peeled

160ml (5½fl oz) double cream

25g (1oz) unsalted butter

salt flakes and freshly ground black pepper

*

I never add too much salt to a sauce if it requires plenty of further reducing. The result will be far too salty due to the flavours becoming concentrated.

Place the chicken breasts between 2 sheets of baking paper and gently flatten the thicker ends using the flat side of a meat mallet. This ensures the breasts are of an even thickness so that they cook evenly.

Choose a deep saucepan that is the right size to allow the chicken breasts to lie snugly in a single layer, while being completely submerged in the poaching liquid. Pour the wine and water into your chosen saucepan and place over a high heat. Add the 3 whole rosemary sprigs and the black peppercorns. Use the back of a knife to smash the garlic cloves before adding them to the pan. Bring to the boil, then add the chicken breasts. Cover with a lid and reduce the heat to medium.

Simmer for 20 minutes, then use a temperature probe to check the thickest piece of one of the breasts. Once the probe reads 70°C (158°F), you can remove the chicken from the pan and set aside on a plate, covered with foil to keep warm. (The temperature that is considered safe for chicken is 72°C/162°F, but if you keep the probe in, you will notice that the chicken continues to rise in temperature while resting. By removing it from the poaching liquid 2 degrees 'early', we avoid overcooking and achieve delicious, succulent chicken.)

Strain the poaching liquid into a smaller, clean saucepan and discard the solids. Place the saucepan over a medium–high heat and cook until reduced to about 60ml (4 tablespoons) of very concentrated liquid. Reduce the heat to low and pour in the cream, whisking well to prevent the sauce splitting. Add the butter, a little a time, whisking between each addition, until the sauce is well-emulsified and thick enough to coat the back of a spoon. Stir in the finely chopped rosemary.

Slice the rested chicken breasts and serve with the sauce. Season with salt flakes (if needed) and freshly ground black pepper.

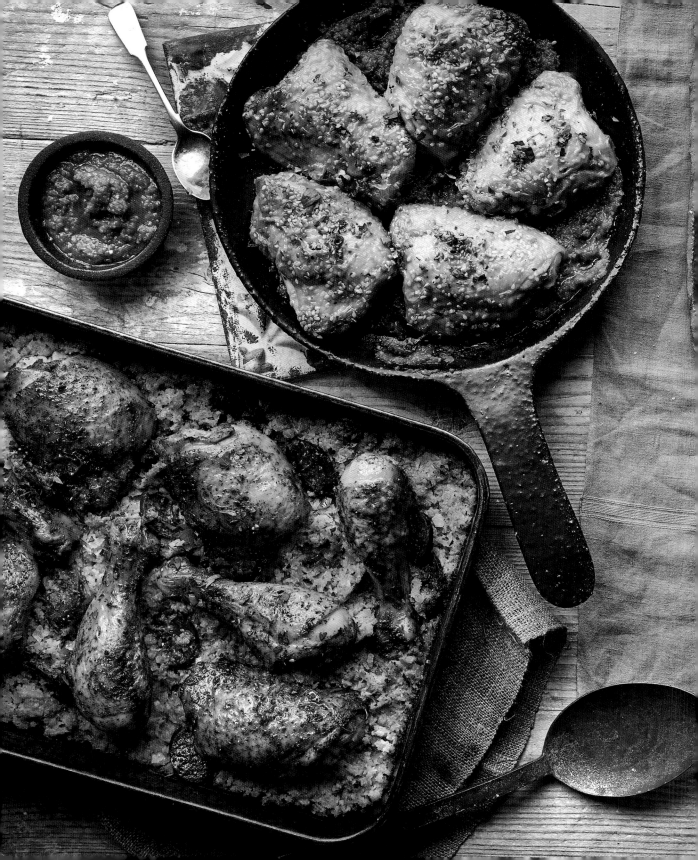

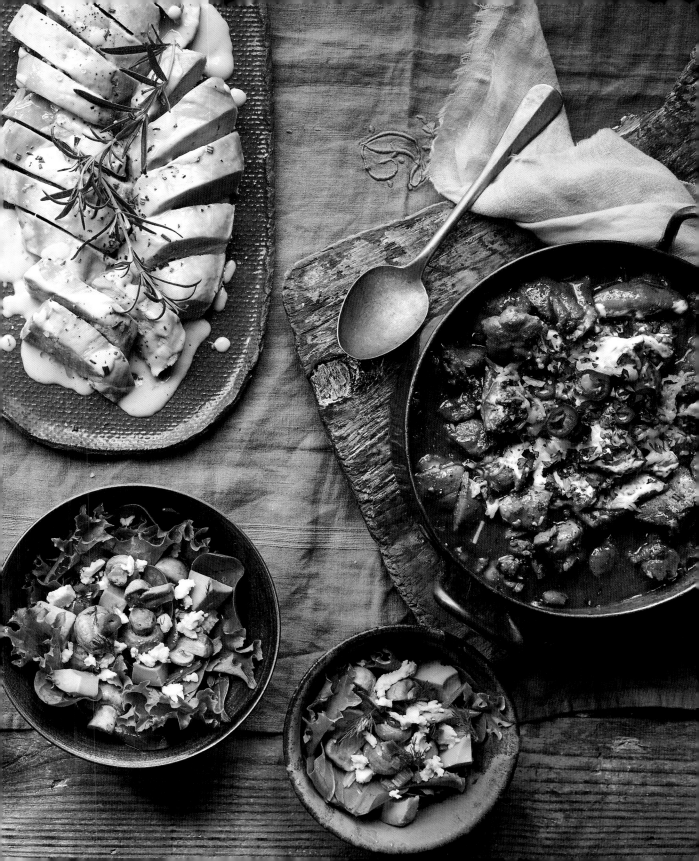

Chicken & Chorizo Bake

This is a scrumptious family chicken dish with flavours of caramelised onion, garlic and paprika. My husband loves the addition of spicy chorizo, which adds a fabulous little kick! Unlike the other recipes, where I have stuck to moderate protein as keto suggests, I think here you will want an extra drumstick as it's so moreish. A friend once told me that this dish 'feels like a hug', and I could not agree more! *Pictured on page 74.*

4 SERVINGS | **15m** PREP TIME | **40m** COOK TIME

CALORIES 608 | CARBOHYDRATES 6.8G | PROTEIN 47G | FAT 43G

8 chicken pieces (thighs and drumsticks), skin on, approx. 1.2kg (2lb 10oz) total weight

½ tablespoon smoked paprika

600g (1lb 5oz) cauliflower florets

30g (1oz) unsalted butter

½ onion, finely chopped

3 garlic cloves, finely chopped

100g (3½oz) best-quality spicy chorizo ring, sliced

salt flakes, salt and freshly ground black pepper

generous handful of fresh flat-leaf parsley leaves, finely chopped, to garnish

Preheat the oven to 200°C/180°C fan/400°F/gas mark 6.

Remove the chicken from its packaging and pat dry with paper towels. Place in a large bowl and scatter over the smoked paprika. Season with salt and freshly ground black pepper, then get stuck in with clean hands and massage the seasoning into the chicken. Arrange the pieces, skin-side up, in a large, deep roasting dish and bake for 20 minutes.

Meanwhile, place the cauliflower in a food processor and blitz until it resembles coarse breadcrumbs. (If you are using a mini food processor, this is best done in 2 or 3 batches.)

Melt the butter in a large non-stick frying pan or wok over a medium heat. Add the onion and cook for 5–6 minutes until it softens and starts to caramelise. Add the garlic and continue to cook for a further 1 minute. Tip in all the cauliflower 'rice' and increase the heat to high, stirring continuously for 3–4 minutes until the cauliflower softens. Stir in the sliced chorizo and remove the pan from the heat

Once the chicken has been in the oven for 20 minutes, take the roasting dish out of the oven and use tongs to remove the chicken pieces, setting them aside on a plate. Add the cauliflower mixture to the roasting dish, stirring it into all the rendered fat and chicken juices present. Return the chicken pieces to the roasting dish, nestling them in among the cauli 'rice' mixture. Return to the oven for another 15–18 minutes until the chicken has safely cooked through. If in doubt, use a thermometer probe to check the thickest part of a thigh. It should read 72°C (162°F).

Season with salt flakes (if needed) and freshly ground black pepper. Scatter over the chopped parsley to finish. Yum!

Chicken

with Sesame & Chilli Sauce

I am a huge fan of chicken thighs (especially on keto, where I can enjoy that crispy, heavenly skin, guilt-free!). These sesame-scattered chicken thighs are served with a delicious sauce made up of rendered fat, chillies, toasted sesame oil and a few other bits. A good scattering of chopped coriander will finish this easy dish perfectly. Serve with your favourite greens on the side. *Pictured on page 74.*

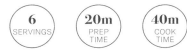

6 SERVINGS | **20m** PREP TIME | **40m** COOK TIME

CALORIES 432 | CARBOHYDRATES 1.5G | PROTEIN 30G | FAT 34G

6 large chicken thighs, skin on (approx. 1kg/2lb 4oz total weight)

2 tablespoons sesame seeds

2–3 red chillies, deseeded and roughly chopped (see Tip)

½ red onion, roughly chopped

3 garlic cloves, roughly chopped

1½ tablespoons double-concentrate tomato purée

60ml (4 tablespoons) water

1 teaspoon rice wine vinegar

1 tablespoon toasted sesame oil

salt flakes and salt

small handful of fresh coriander leaves, finely chopped, to garnish

*

If you like things super spicy, do not discard all the seeds from the chillies when preparing them: the seeds are where the heat lies!

Preheat the oven to 200°C/180°C fan/400°F/gas mark 6.

Season the undersides of the chicken thighs with salt, then place, skin-side up, on a baking tray. Scatter over the sesame seeds and bake for 30–35 minutes until the skins are golden and crispy and the chicken has safely cooked through. If in doubt, use a thermometer probe to check the thickest part of a thigh. It should read 72°C (162°F).

Meanwhile, place the chillies, red onion, garlic, tomato purée and water in a mini food processor. Blitz until smooth, stopping to scrape down the sides of the bowl. Transfer the mixture to a small saucepan and place over a medium–high heat. Cook for 10–12 minutes to cook out any raw flavours. Stir in the rice wine vinegar and return to the food processor for now.

Once the chicken thighs are cooked through and their skins are crispy, remove them from the tray and set aside to keep warm. Pour all the fat and juices from the tray into the food processor, over the cooked chilli and tomato paste. Add the sesame oil and blitz together to form a fairly smooth, emulsified sauce. Return the sauce to the small saucepan to warm through if you feel it needs it before serving.

Serve the chicken with the sauce and scatter over the chopped coriander. Season with salt flakes if needed.

Rib-eye Steaks

with a Baked Mushroom & Bay Sauce

4 SERVINGS   **10m** PREP TIME   **45m** COOK TIME

This dish was one of my experiments that turned out simply perfect! The mushrooms are flash-fried for caramelisation, then baked in the oven in a garlic and bay-infused cream. Dried bay leaves offer a much better flavour, so don't worry about trying to source fresh ones. The mushroom sauce is so intoxicating when smothered over a juicy rib-eye – it is well worth the time and effort. Mark says this dish is 'restaurant-quality'... High praise, but I'll take it!

CALORIES 1088 | CARBOHYDRATES 6.1G | PROTEIN 62G | FAT 91G

30g (1oz) unsalted butter

4 rib-eye steaks (approx. 220g/7¾oz each)

salt flakes and freshly ground black pepper

For the baked mushroom sauce

60g (2¼oz) unsalted butter

450g (1lb) mushrooms, halved (larger ones quartered)

2 garlic cloves, finely sliced

300ml (10fl oz) double cream

3–4 dried bay leaves

30g (1oz) Parmesan cheese, finely grated

salt and ground white pepper

Preheat the oven to 200°C/180°C fan/400°F/gas mark 6.

Begin by making the sauce. You will need to fry the mushrooms in batches. Heat a third of the butter in a large non-stick frying pan over a high heat. Once it is foaming, add half the mushrooms and fry for 3–4 minutes until they start to turn golden and caramelise. There should be no moisture left in the pan. Remove and set aside on a plate. Repeat with another third of the butter and the remaining mushrooms and transfer these to the plate as well. Season lightly with salt.

Add the remaining butter to the pan, along with the garlic. Reduce the heat to low and cook for 1-2 minutes until the garlic has softened. Pour the cream into the pan and add the bay leaves, increasing the heat to medium–high so the mixture starts to simmer.

Return the mushrooms to the pan and cook for 2–3 minutes, scraping down the sides of the pan as the cream reduces and infuses. Stir through the Parmesan and season with salt and white pepper. Transfer the entire mixture (including the bay leaves) to an ovenproof baking dish measuring approximately 15 x 15cm (6 x 6in). Bake for 25–28 minutes, rotating the dish halfway through.

Meanwhile, prepare the steaks. Melt the butter in a large frying pan over a high heat and add the steaks. Cook until done to your liking, then remove and set aside to rest for 10 minutes. Season with salt flakes and plenty of freshly ground black pepper.

Remove the mushroom bake from the oven and discard the bay leaves. You can spoon the mushrooms over the top of the steaks as a sauce, or you could slice the steaks and combine them with the mushrooms, creating a rich, beefy dish to enjoy over courgetti or cauliflower mash.

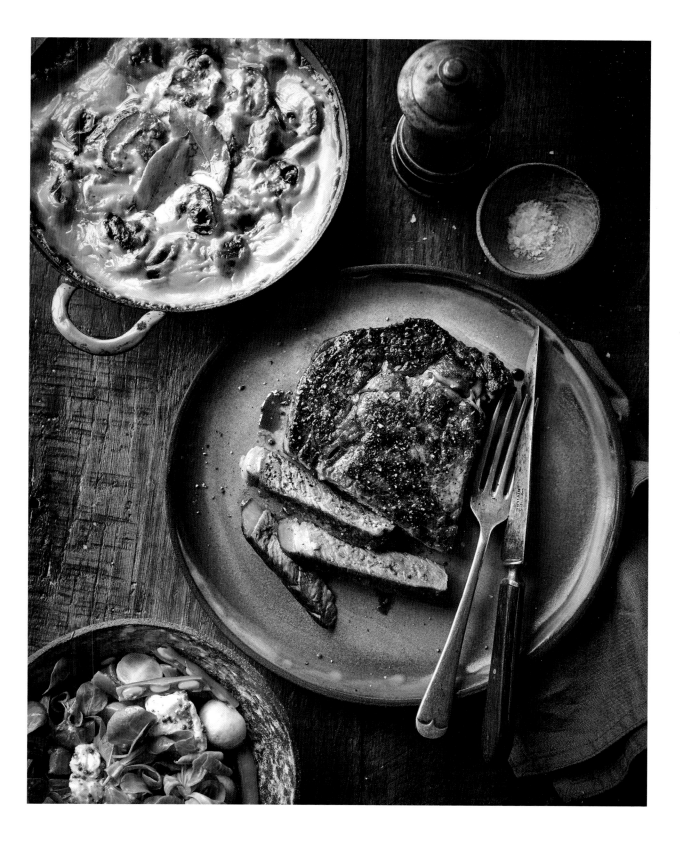

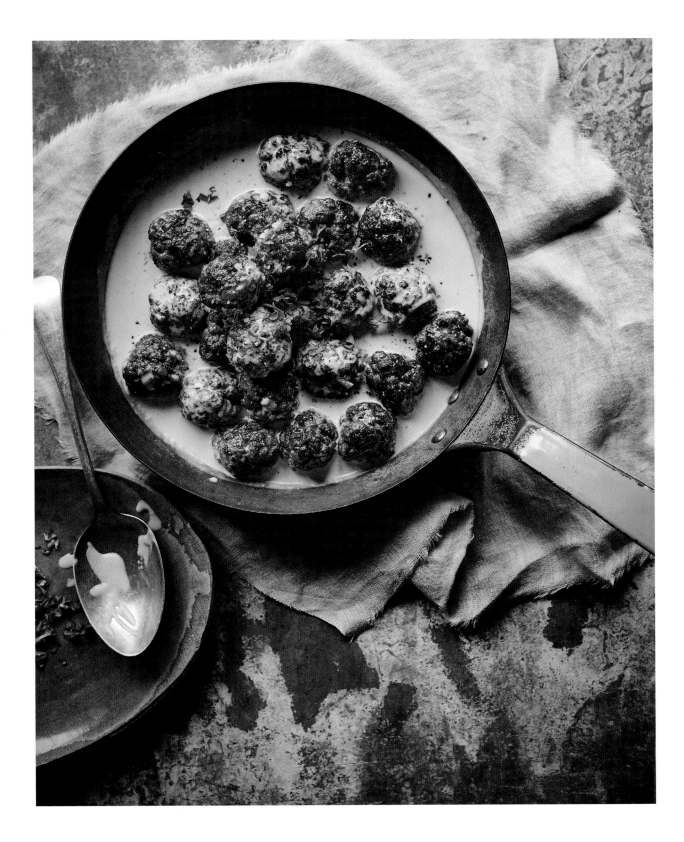

Creamy Swedish Meatballs

This is my version of Swedish meatballs, where small, fragrantly spiced meatballs are served in a deliciously creamy sauce boasting a hint of mustard and bay. It will have you forgetting all about meatballs marinara! Browning the meatballs over a high heat achieves the best caramelisation, and then you can gently finish them in the oven while you make the sauce. Enjoy over your favourite base, like cauliflower mash or buttered courgette noodles.

 4 SERVINGS   **20m** PREP TIME   **35m** COOK TIME

CALORIES 708 | CARBOHYDRATES 4.7G | PROTEIN 35G | FAT 60G

For the meatballs

300g (10½oz) minced beef, 20 per cent fat

300g (10½oz) minced pork, 12 per cent fat

1 tablespoon ground chia seeds

2 teaspoons ground allspice

¼ teaspoon ground nutmeg

2 tablespoons unsalted butter

salt and ground white pepper

For the sauce

200ml (7fl oz) double cream

100g (3½oz) soured cream

2 teaspoons Dijon mustard

½ onion, finely chopped

2 garlic cloves, finely chopped

1 dried bay leaf

250ml (9fl oz) best-quality beef stock, warm

salt flakes and freshly ground black pepper

small handful of fresh flat-leaf or curly parsley leaves, finely chopped, to garnish

Preheat the oven to 150°C/130°C fan/300°F/gas mark 2 and line a baking tray with baking paper.

Combine all the meatball ingredients except the butter in a bowl and season generously with salt and ground white pepper. Use a dessertspoon to form approximately 26 small, compact meatballs.

Cook in 2 batches. Melt half the butter in a large non-stick frying pan over a high heat and add half the meatballs. Fry until browned on the outsides, using a spoon to gently turn them over. Once they are browned, use a slotted spoon to remove them from the pan and set aside on the prepared baking tray, leaving the fat in the pan. Repeat with the remaining butter and meatballs. Transfer to the oven for 15–17 minutes so they can finish cooking through.

Meanwhile, make the sauce. In a bowl, whisk together the double cream, soured cream and mustard. Set aside.

Place the frying pan you used for the meatballs over a medium heat and add the onion. Gently cook for 5–6 minutes until softened, then add the garlic and cook for a further 1 minute until softened. Add the bay leaf and pour in the stock. Increase the heat to high and bring to the boil. Continue to cook over a high heat for 10–12 minutes until the stock reduces to a very thick consistency.

Reduce the heat to medium–low and pour in the whisked cream mixture, stirring well. Allow the sauce to gently reduce and infuse.

By this time, your meatballs should be ready to add to the sauce and serve. Pick out the bay leaf and discard, and season the mixture with salt flakes and freshly ground black pepper. Garnish with parsley to add a fresh element and serve with your chosen base.

Show-stopping Beef Stir-fry

Stir-fries are the perfect midweek meal when you want minimal washing up. Asian stir-fries often have brown sugar added to balance out the salty soy, so I simply reach for a little sugar-free 'maple' syrup instead, and also opt for tamari (gluten-free soy sauce). You will notice I prepare the elements in stages, ensuring each ingredient is respected and prepared exactly as it should be to ensure the perfect outcome. This can be enjoyed over courgetti or konjac (shirataki) noodles, but I love it with my Egg-fried 'Rice' (page 107).

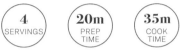

4 SERVINGS | **20m** PREP TIME | **35m** COOK TIME

CALORIES 552 | CARBOHYDRATES 6.6G | PROTEIN 54G | FAT 34G

170g (6oz) long-stem broccoli, trimmed (trimmed weight)

700g (1lb 9oz) rump steak, patted dry with paper towels and sliced along the grain into thin strips

1 teaspoon ground coriander

1 teaspoon ground ginger

3 tablespoons unflavoured coconut oil

25g (1oz) fresh root ginger, peeled and finely minced

3 garlic cloves, finely chopped

1 lemongrass stalk, finely chopped (discard the hard outer layer)

1 red chilli, finely chopped, plus optional extra chilli slices, to serve

1 red pepper, finely sliced

200g (7oz) mushrooms, thickly sliced

3 tablespoons tamari (gluten-free soy sauce)

1 tablespoon sugar-free 'maple' syrup

1 tablespoon toasted sesame oil

juice of 1 lime

salt

small handful of fresh coriander leaves, finely chopped, to garnish

2 teaspoons sesame seeds, to garnish (optional)

Bring a saucepan of salted water to a rapid boil over a high heat. Add the broccoli and cook for 2 minutes, then drain and set aside.

Place the sliced steak in a large bowl and season lightly with salt. Scatter over the ground coriander and ground ginger and toss well to evenly coat the pieces. The steaks will appear 'dry' when tossed in this spice mix, which will make for excellent flash-frying.

Heat 1 tablespoon of the coconut oil in a large non-stick frying pan or wok over a very high heat. Stir-fry the beef slices, working in batches, for 1–2 minutes per batch until they are golden and caramelised on the outside. The high heat of the pan will quickly brown the meat, ensuring a lovely caramelisation without overcooking. After each batch, remove the beef slices from the pan or wok and set aside in a large bowl.

Reduce the heat to low and add another 1 tablespoon coconut oil to the pan. Add the finely chopped ginger, garlic, lemongrass and chilli. Cook, stirring occasionally, until the mixture softens completely – this can take up to 10 minutes. Pour this mixture over the steaks and stir.

Return the empty pan to a medium heat and add the remaining coconut oil. Add the red pepper and stir-fry for about 2 minutes. Once softened, increase the heat to high and add the mushrooms. Cook for 3–4 minutes, stirring regularly to caramelise the mushrooms beautifully. Reduce the heat to medium and return the beef mixture to the pan, along with the broccoli. Add the tamari and sugar-free 'maple' syrup. Warm everything through and stir well to coat in the lovely sauce. Just before serving, stir through the sesame oil and squeeze over the fresh lime juice. Serve, garnished with the chopped coriander and sliced chillies and sesame seeds, if using.

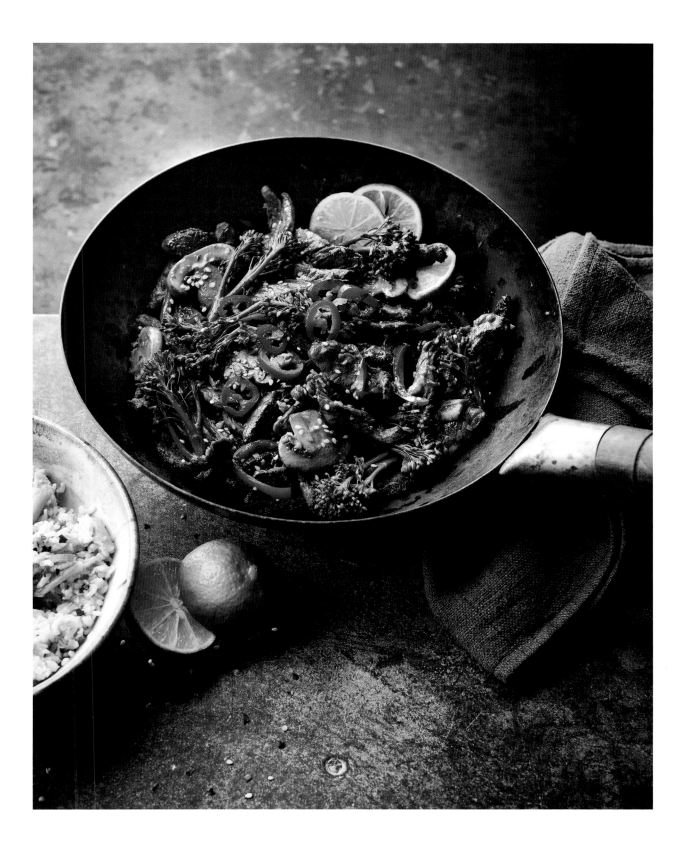

South African 'Bobotie'

I simply had to showcase one of South Africa's traditional dishes: Bobotie. This is my version, where I have changed some of the more traditional ingredients to make it more low-carb friendly. In a nutshell, this bake features a fragrant, spicy mince with little hints of sweetness, covered in a savoury 'custard' to which I have added cream cheese and turmeric. This dish is packed with interesting flavours from my beloved home country: please try it!

6 SERVINGS | **20m** PREP TIME | **1hr10** COOK TIME

CALORIES 556 | CARBOHYDRATES 4.5G | PROTEIN 29G | FAT 46G

For the spiced beef

2 teaspoons lard or ghee

½ onion, finely chopped

2 garlic cloves, finely chopped

1½ tablespoons medium curry powder

1 teaspoon ground ginger

¼ teaspoon ground cloves

750g (1lb 10oz) minced beef, 20 per cent fat

250ml (9fl oz) best-quality beef stock

20g (¾oz) dried cranberries, chopped very small (see Tip)

2 tablespoons ground chia seeds

1 tablespoon powdered erythritol, sifted

salt and freshly ground black pepper

For the turmeric egg topping

3 large eggs

180ml (6fl oz) double cream

45g (1½oz) full-fat cream cheese

¾ teaspoon ground turmeric

3 dried bay leaves

10g (¼oz) flaked almonds, toasted

ground white pepper

Preheat the oven to 200°C/180°C fan/400°F/gas mark 6.

Melt the lard or ghee in a large non-stick frying pan over a medium heat. Add the onion and cook for 6–7 minutes until it softens and starts to caramelise. Add the garlic, curry powder and spices, cooking for a few seconds and stirring. Tip in the minced beef and increase the heat to high, breaking up the mince with your spoon. Cook for 8–10 minutes until the beef is evenly browned. Pour in the stock and continue to cook over this high heat, stirring, until you are left with a chunky mixture completely free of excess moisture. This can take 10–12 minutes. Remove from the heat and stir in the cranberries, ground chia seeds and erythritol. Taste and adjust the seasoning generously with salt and freshly ground black pepper.

Transfer the mixture to a deep ovenproof dish (the one I used was 18 x 24cm/7 x 9½in and 5cm/2in deep). Compact the mixture down, ensuring you leave space for the egg topping later. Cover with foil and make several holes in the foil with a cocktail stick. Bake for 20 minutes.

Meanwhile, prepare the egg topping. In a large bowl, simply whisk together the eggs, cream, cream cheese and turmeric until there are no lumps. Season with salt and ground white pepper, then set aside.

Remove the dish from the oven and discard the foil. You will notice the mixture looks very greasy, so lay a sheet of good-quality paper towel on top to soak up the unnecessary grease. Pour the seasoned creamy egg mixture over the top of the beef and place the 3 bay leaves on top. Return to the oven for 15 minutes, then turn off the oven, leaving the dish inside for a further 5 minutes to gently finish cooking in the residual heat. Scatter over the toasted almonds before tucking in!

*

Store-bought dried cranberries often contain extra sugar. Chopping them small makes a little go a long way, ensuring the little bites of sweetness characteristic of a bobotie.

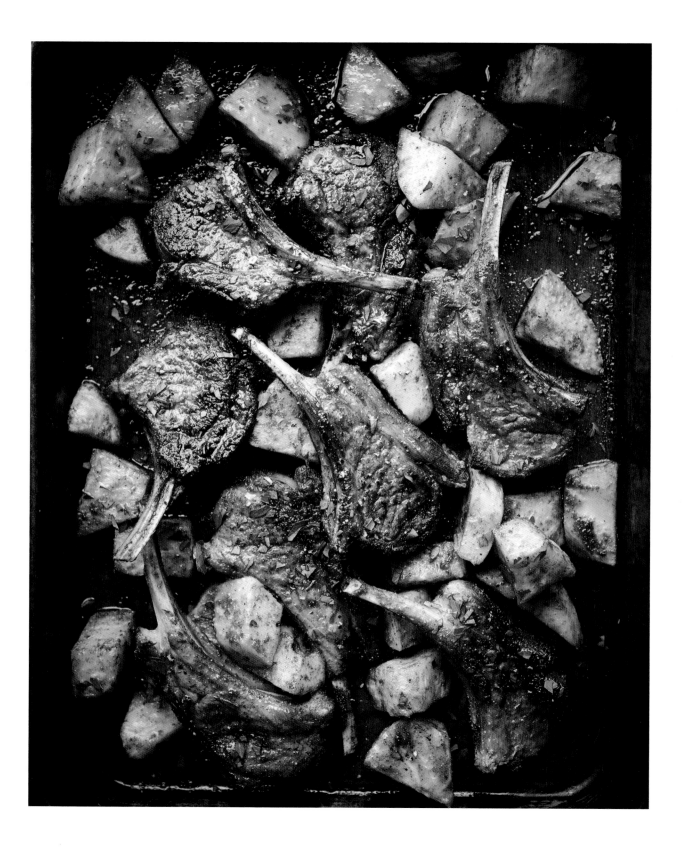

Spicy Lamb Traybake

with Celeriac Roasties

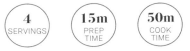

Spicy and sweet, these celeriac roasties hit the spot as the perfect side dish if you are missing potatoes on your low-carb journey. I flavour the melted butter with an interesting combination of spices before pouring it over partially cooked celeriac chunks. These then get roasted alongside spiced lamb cutlets (you could also use chops). This is a winner – and just lovely with your favourite greens on the side.

CALORIES 599 | CARBOHYDRATES 4.9G | PROTEIN 26G | FAT 51G

8 lamb cutlets or chops (approx. 900g/2lb total weight)

1 teaspoon ground cumin

1 teaspoon ground coriander

salt, salt flakes and freshly ground black pepper

small handful of fresh flat-leaf parsley leaves, finely chopped, to garnish

For the celeriac roasties

500g (1lb 2oz) celeriac, peeled and cut into 4cm (1½in) chunks (trimmed weight)

25g (1oz) unsalted butter

1 teaspoon ground cumin

1 teaspoon ground coriander

1 teaspoon cayenne pepper

salt

Preheat the oven to 200°C/180°C fan/400°F/gas mark 6.

To make the celeriac roasties, bring a large saucepan of salted water to the boil and boil the celeriac chunks for 10–12 minutes to partially cook. Drain in a colander and allow to steam until completely dry. It helps if you spread them out on a tray lined with paper towels. Once dry, place them in a large bowl.

Meanwhile, melt the butter in a small saucepan over a medium heat and whisk in the cumin, coriander and cayenne pepper. Pour this flavoured butter into the bowl of celeriac and toss gently to evenly coat the pieces. Spread them out on a large baking tray and bake for 10–12 minutes.

Season the lamb cutlets or chops with the cumin, coriander and some salt. Once the celeriac chunks have had their initial bake, remove the baking tray from the oven and add the lamb cutlets or chops, nestling them in among the celeriac. Bake for 20–25 minutes until the lamb is cooked through to your liking and the celeriac has sufficiently softened.

Serve immediately, seasoned with salt flakes and freshly ground black pepper. Scatter with finely chopped parsley.

Lamb Rogan Josh

This is a fresh and beautifully spiced curry featuring my favourite red meat. Enjoy this comforting dish with your favourite low-carb base, such as a cauliflower 'rice' cooked with a little ground turmeric. I like to serve this with my delicious Cumin Flatbreads (page 110) as pictured (not included in the macros). Do not omit the swirl of yogurt and scattering of fresh coriander before serving, as this finishes off the dish perfectly.

4 SERVINGS | **20m** PREP TIME | **1hr20** COOK TIME

CALORIES 688 | CARBOHYDRATES 8.7G | PROTEIN 43G | FAT 53G

400g (14oz) can chopped tomatoes

120ml (4fl oz) water

1 tablespoon double-concentrate tomato purée

3 tablespoons ghee

900g (2lb) diced lamb shoulder

½ onion, finely chopped

3 garlic cloves, finely chopped

15g (½oz) fresh root ginger, peeled and minced

1 cinnamon stick

2 teaspoons ground cumin

2 teaspoons ground coriander

2 teaspoons chilli powder

2 teaspoons paprika

1 teaspoon cardamom pods, lightly crushed

pinch of ground cloves

80g (2¾oz) full-fat plain yogurt

salt flakes and freshly ground black pepper

small handful of fresh coriander leaves, finely chopped, to garnish

Place the chopped tomatoes in a mini food processor along with the water and tomato purée. Blitz well until smooth, then set aside.

Cook the lamb in 3 batches. Heat 1 tablespoon of the ghee in a large non-stick frying pan over a high heat. Add a third of the lamb pieces and cook for 3–4 minutes until browned and caramelised. Remove with a slotted spoon and set aside in a bowl. Repeat with the remaining ghee and lamb until all the lamb is cooked, then set aside.

Return the pan to the hob – there should be plenty of fat left in the pan from cooking the lamb. Reduce the heat to medium, add the onion and cook for 5–6 minutes until softened, all the while scraping the bottom of the pan to loosen any bits of stuck meat (this is flavour!). Add the garlic and ginger and cook for a further 1 minute until the mixture starts to caramelise.

Now add the cinnamon stick, cumin, coriander, chilli powder, paprika, cardamom pods and ground cloves. Stir well, then pour in the tomato mixture and bring to the boil. Reduce the heat to low and return the lamb to the pan, along with any resting juices from the bowl. Cover with a lid and leave to simmer gently for 1 hour. I always remove the lid in the last 10–12 minutes to ensure the mixture thickens sufficiently. Taste and adjust the seasoning using salt flakes and freshly ground black pepper.

Just before serving, stir through the yogurt and scatter over the finely chopped coriander.

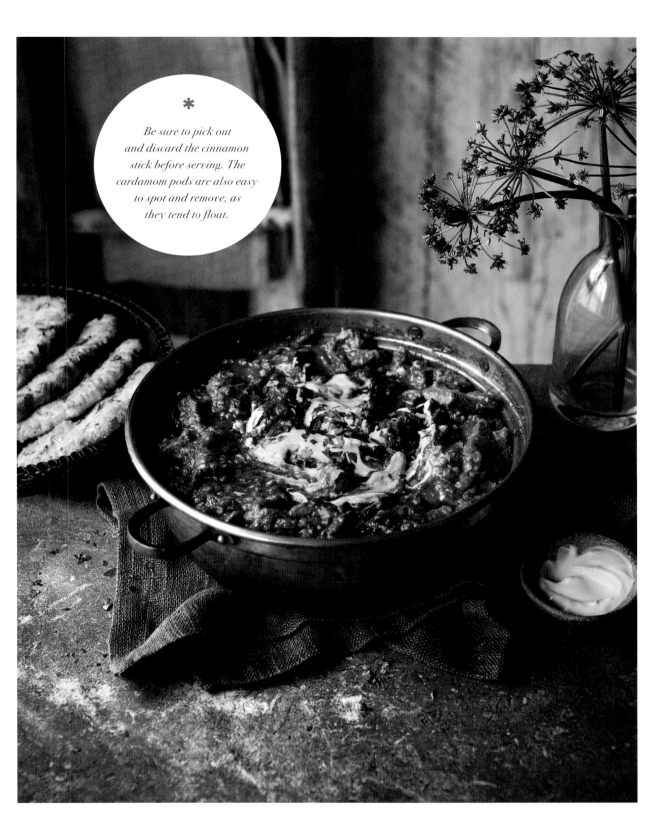

*

Be sure to pick out and discard the cinnamon stick before serving. The cardamom pods are also easy to spot and remove, as they tend to float.

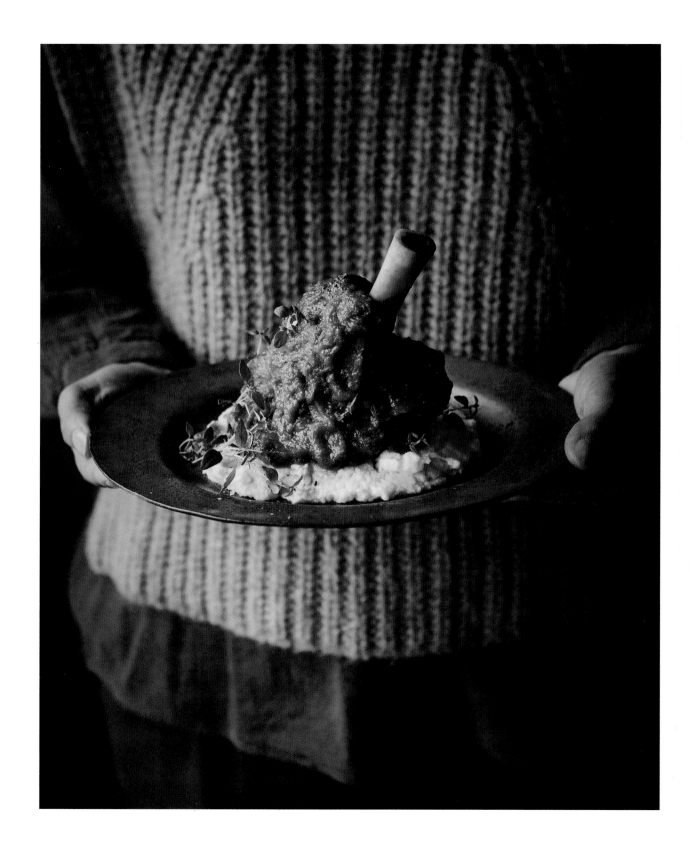

Lamb Shanks

with Herby Tomato 'Gravy'

The meat from one lamb shank could easily feed two people, making this a lovely option to slow-cook on a lazy Sunday for visiting guests and family, leaving you with only one concern: which lucky four get to suck out the marrow? The slow-cooking part can be made in a large slow-cooker, but the browning of the elements and the reduction of the sauce must be done on the hob. These shanks are delicious served over Cheesy Celeriac Mash (page 111) as pictured, or with my Mini Rosemary Rolls (page 108) to mop up the yummy sauce.

CALORIES 422 | CARBOHYDRATES 4.2G | PROTEIN 40G | FAT 27G

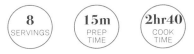

8 SERVINGS | **15m** PREP TIME | **2hr40** COOK TIME

1 tablespoon lard or ghee

4 lamb shanks (approx. 1.6kg/3lb 8oz total weight)

½ onion, finely chopped

1 celery stick, finely chopped

3 garlic cloves, finely chopped

2 teaspoons dried thyme

1 teaspoon paprika

60ml (4 tablespoons) red wine

400g (14oz) chopped tomatoes, canned or fresh

2 tablespoons double-concentrate tomato purée

500ml (18fl oz) best-quality beef stock

2 dried bay leaves

2 fresh rosemary sprigs, needles picked and finely chopped

salt, salt flakes and freshly ground black pepper

fresh thyme leaves, to garnish

Melt the lard or ghee in a large, deep non-stick frying pan over a high heat. Lightly salt the lamb shanks, then add them to the pan and brown on all sides for 4–5 minutes until golden and caramelised. Their shape makes this step a little tricky, but do the best you can as this browning process improves the overall flavour. Remove and set aside on a plate.

There should be plenty of fat left in the pan. Reduce the heat to medium and add the onion and celery. Cook for 5–6 minutes until softened, then add the garlic, dried thyme and paprika and cook for 1 minute more before adding the red wine. Cook until all the wine evaporates, then add the chopped tomatoes, tomato purée, beef stock, bay leaves and rosemary. Bring the mixture to the boil, then reduce the heat to low. Return the lamb shanks to the pan, nestling them in together in an even layer. Partially cover with a lid and leave to simmer gently for 2 hours. Every now and then, check in on the shanks, turning them gently and spooning over the sauce, scraping the sides of the pan down with a silicone spatula.

After 2 hours, gently remove the shanks from the pan and set aside, covered with foil to keep warm. Pick out and discard the bay leaves from the tomato mixture, then use a hand blender to blitz the sauce in the pan until smooth. If the sauce is too thick, let it down with a dash of water. On the other hand, if it's not a nice, thick consistency, increase the heat to medium and cook until reduced.

Serve the lamb shanks with the sauce poured over the top and season with salt flakes and freshly ground black pepper. Scatter over freshly picked thyme leaves for additional flavour.

Kielbasa Sausage Rolls

These sausage rolls are fabulously rich and remind me of ones I had growing up in South Africa. They are only an occasional indulgence of ours as I use kielbasa (a smoked Polish sausage found in the deli meat aisle). Kielbasa is very low in carbs, but it is rightly considered 'dirty' keto (see pages 5–6)! This recipe makes two indulgent rolls – it's likely you may not even finish one in one sitting. Try it with the optional tomato relish (not included in the macros), which does a great job of cutting through the richness!

2 SERVINGS | **25m** PREP TIME | **1hr30** CHILL TIME | **25m** COOK TIME

CALORIES 1031 | CARBOHYDRATES 8.1G | PROTEIN 53G | FAT 86G

80g (2¾oz) almond flour

1 teaspoon baking powder

1 teaspoon garlic powder

140g (5oz) extra-mature full-fat Cheddar cheese, grated

50g (1¾oz) full-fat cream cheese

2 small–medium eggs

280g (10oz) kielbasa (smoked Polish sausage)

1 teaspoon sesame seeds

salt

For the tomato relish (optional)

2 tomatoes, finely chopped

1 red chilli, finely chopped

2 teaspoons no-added-sugar ketchup

*

It is important that the dough is chilled at all times, so do not leave your prepared rolls at room temperature for too long before baking, or the dough may slide away in the oven.

In a food processor, mix together the almond flour, baking powder, garlic powder and a generous pinch of salt. Place the Cheddar in a wide-bottomed, microwave-safe bowl and microwave on high for 60–90 seconds until melted. Carefully remove from the microwave and stir in the cream cheese, then tip the whole lot into the food processor with the dry ingredients and blitz.

Add 1 of the eggs and whizz again until the mixture forms a sticky dough. Spread the dough out on to a long sheet of baking paper and cover with a second sheet. Roll the dough out into a rectangle measuring approximately 20 x 25cm (8 x 10in). Chill for 1 hour 30 minutes.

Preheat the oven to 200°C/180°C fan/400°F/gas mark 6 and line a baking tray with a clean sheet of baking paper.

Remove the dough from the fridge and peel off the top layer of baking paper. Neaten up the edges of the rectangle, then divide it in half. Cut the bottom sheet of baking paper in half as well, so you can work with each piece individually. Cut the sausage into 2 even-sized pieces (each approximately 14cm/5½in long) and place 1 sausage on each piece of dough. Roll the dough around the sausage, peeling off the baking paper as you go. Place the sausage rolls on the prepared baking tray. Working quickly, whisk the second egg in a small bowl to make an egg wash, and brush this over the sausage rolls. Scatter over the sesame seeds and bake for 20–25 minutes, rotating the tray halfway through.

If you'd like to make the fresh tomato relish, simply mix all the ingredients together in a small bowl. Serve the sausage rolls warm with the relish on the side (if using).

*

If you prefer a 'cleaner'
sausage roll, use whichever
sausages you are more
comfortable enjoying – but
they must be precooked.

Kielbasa & Cabbage Soup

For a soup made with a handful of simple ingredients, this really packs a punch when it comes to flavour. This is an utterly filthy keto soup – please see pages 5–6 for why processed meats like kielbasa (smoked Polish sausage) are best left for occasional consumption only, despite being low in carbohydrates. *Pictured on page 93.*

4 SERVINGS | **10m** PREP TIME | **20m** COOK TIME

CALORIES 244 | CARBOHYDRATES 5.9G | PROTEIN 16G | FAT 16G

2 teaspoons ghee or lard

4 spring onions, green and white parts separated, sliced

400g (14oz) Savoy cabbage, thinly sliced

1 teaspoon smoked paprika

240g (8½oz) kielbasa (smoked Polish sausage), sliced

1.2 litres (2 pints) best-quality chicken stock

1 dried bay leaf

Heat the ghee or lard in a large saucepan over a medium heat. Add the white parts of the spring onions, along with the cabbage and smoked paprika. Cook, stirring continuously, for 5 minutes until the cabbage starts to soften.

Add the sliced sausage to the pan and pour in the chicken stock, then add the bay leaf and bring to the boil. Reduce the heat to low, cover with a lid and simmer gently for 14–15 minutes to allow all those flavours to hang around and get to know each other.

Pick out and discard the bay leaf, then divide the soup between 4 warm bowls. Serve garnished with the green parts of the spring onions. So simple, so yummy!

*

I love using the soft, inner leaves of Savoy cabbage. You can use regular cabbage here, but it will need much longer on the heat to soften sufficiently.

Prosciutto & Mozzarella Salad

2 SERVINGS   **10m** PREP TIME

This great salad can be served as a side option at your next *braai* (barbecue), but there is sufficient protein in there (from the mozzarella and prosciutto) to make it a perfectly filling option for a quick lunch. I use a little sugar-free 'maple' syrup in the dressing, which balances out the salty prosciutto just wonderfully. You should always dress your salad just before serving to prevent the salad leaves wilting, so keep your dressing in a separate little container if you want to take this to work with you. *Pictured on page 104.*

CALORIES 422 | CARBOHYDRATES 1.9G | PROTEIN 25G | FAT 35G

100g (3½oz) mixed baby salad leaves

120g (4¼oz) best-quality prosciutto

70g (2½oz) baby mozzarella balls (pearls), drained well (see Tip)

4–5 fresh basil leaves, thinly sliced

freshly ground black pepper

For the dressing

3 tablespoons olive oil

1 tablespoon red wine vinegar

1 teaspoon Dijon mustard

1 teaspoon sugar-free 'maple' syrup

¼ teaspoon dried oregano

Place the salad leaves in a bowl (or divide between 2 bowls), and arrange the strips of prosciutto over the top. If you like, you could tear the prosciutto strips into smaller pieces. Scatter over the drained mozzarella balls and the shredded basil.

In a small bowl or jug, whisk together all the dressing ingredients, then pour the dressing over the salad just before serving. This salad may not require additional salt due to the saltiness of the prosciutto, but a fresh crack of black pepper would be perfect!

*

If you cannot source the little mozzarella balls, simply tear a large fresh ball of mozzarella into smaller pieces.

Garlic Pork Ribs

that Fall Off the Bone!

Once you've tried this method, you will never want to prepare your ribs in any other way! These literally fall off the bone. I slow-cook the racks in air-tight parcels of foil at a low temperature for several hours before finishing them in a hot oven or on the *braai* (barbecue) after brushing with the rich and tasty garlic marinade. If you don't want a strong garlic flavour, reduce the amount of garlic paste to 1 teaspoon. If you prefer not to use tamari, coconut aminos is a great alternative. The recipe calls for two racks of pork ribs, shared between four people.

CALORIES 488 | CARBOHYDRATES 2G | PROTEIN 43G | FAT 34G

4 SERVINGS | **5m** PREP TIME | **3hr30** COOK TIME

2 racks of pork ribs, (approx. 900g/2lb total)

90g (3¼oz) no-added-sugar ketchup

2 tablespoons tamari (gluten-free soy sauce)

1 tablespoon olive oil

2 teaspoons Dijon mustard

2 teaspoons store-bought garlic paste

salt flakes and salt

Preheat the oven to 150°C/130°C fan/300°F/gas mark 2.

Use a sharp knife to remove the silver skin from the underside of the racks (see Tip).

Place each rack each on a long piece of strong foil and season with salt. Wrap each rack very tightly in its sheet of foil. The 2 foil parcels should be 100 per cent airtight to ensure that no steam escapes. If in doubt, double wrap. If there is a small hole, wrap again! Place the foil-wrapped parcels on a large baking tray and bake for 3 hours.

Meanwhile, make the marinade by simply combining the ketchup, tamari, olive oil, mustard and garlic paste in a small bowl.

After 3 hours, remove the ribs from the oven, but do not open the foil parcels for at least 20–25 minutes.

To finish, increase the oven temperature to 240°C/220°C fan/475°F/gas mark 9 or prepare your barbecue. Carefully remove the ribs from the foil and brush the racks on both sides with the marinade. Gently place the ribs on a baking tray (or on the barbecue grill) and cook for 7–9 minutes, basting regularly, until the ribs have warmed through again.

Serve with a scattering of salt flakes, if needed.

*

If you choose to finish these on the barbecue, I advise you not to remove the silver skin. The meat might fall right through the grill into your coals – and no one wants such a tragedy!

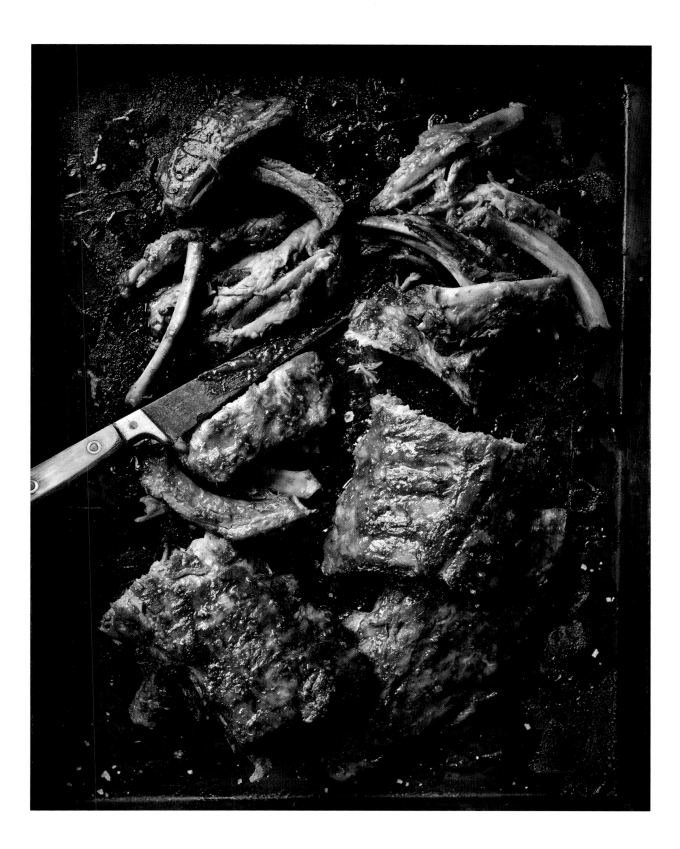

Pork Fillet
with Creamy Leek & Basil Sauce

I first recall making this pork dish when I was only about 22 years old and doing a lousy job at hosting dinner parties for my friends, but I have perfected it over the years. The flavours are beautiful and well worth sharing, even now I'm in my forties! I use pork fillet tenderloins, but it is the creamy leek and basil sauce that steals the show, and it would work just as well with fat, juicy pork chops if you prefer. This is delicious with your favourite greens served alongside.

4 SERVINGS | **20m** PREP TIME | **45m** COOK TIME

CALORIES 485 | CARBOHYDRATES 7.6G | PROTEIN 66G | FAT 21G

2 pork fillets (tenderloins), approx. 450g (1lb) each

1 tablespoon lard or ghee

salt flakes, salt and freshly ground black pepper

For the creamy leek and basil sauce

400g (14oz) chopped tomatoes, canned or fresh

1 tablespoon unsalted butter

3 garlic cloves, finely chopped

200g (7oz) leeks, finely sliced (see Tip)

200ml (7fl oz) best-quality chicken stock

150g (5½oz) soured cream

10–12 fresh basil leaves, thinly sliced

*

Use only the white parts of the leeks, as the green ends are quite tough and can be bitter.

Start with the sauce, as this will take the longest. Blitz the chopped tomatoes in a mini food processor and set aside.

Melt the butter in a large non-stick frying pan or wok over a medium heat. Add the garlic and leeks and fry for 8–10 minutes until softened and just starting to caramelise. Tip in the chicken stock and the blitzed tomatoes and cook for a further 12–15 minutes, allowing the leeks to completely soften and the sauce to thicken. Stir in the soured cream along with most of the shredded basil (reserving a little for garnish). Reduce the heat to low to stay warm while you prepare the pork.

Meanwhile, preheat the oven to 230°C/210°C fan/450°F/gas mark 8.

Season the pork fillets on all sides with salt and a generous amount of freshly ground black pepper. Heat the lard or ghee in a large non-stick pan over a high heat. Add the pork fillets and sear on all sides for 7–8 minutes until golden and caramelised. Transfer them on to a large roasting tray and roast for 12 minutes.

Remove the pork fillets from the oven and cover tightly with foil. Allow to rest for 10 minutes before slicing.

Serve the sliced pork with the sauce. Season with salt flakes (only if needed) before scattering over the remaining basil to garnish.

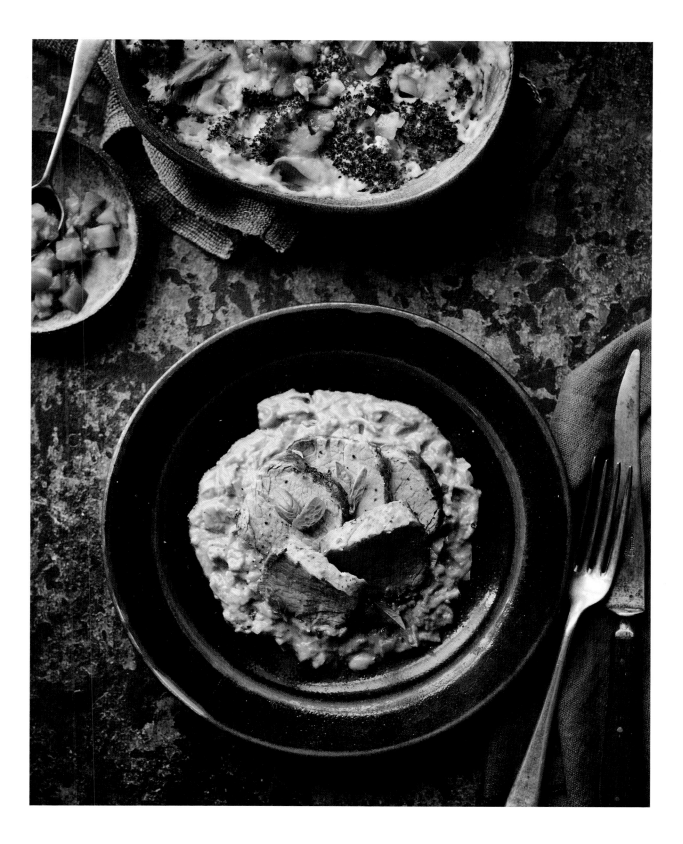

Sausages
with Turmeric Creamed Spinach

I love the sensational 'warm' flavours in this turmeric creamed spinach, which is baked along with caramelised porkies. I only use 1 teaspoon of turmeric (which has so many wonderful properties), but a little goes a long way, and turmeric remains the dominant flavour. Please do not skip the pickled red onion garnish – it adds a delicious, acidic element which finishes this rich and creamy dish to perfection. The recipe is very 'saucy', so it's ideal served over something like cooked, seasoned cauliflower 'rice' or mash.

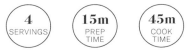

CALORIES 621 | CARBOHYDRATES 5.4G | PROTEIN 23G | FAT 56G

4 SERVINGS   **15m** PREP TIME   **45m** COOK TIME

8 gluten-free pork sausages

2 teaspoons lard or ghee

3 garlic cloves, finely chopped

230g (8¼oz) baby spinach

160ml (5½fl oz) double cream

70g (2½oz) soured cream

60g (2¼oz) full-fat cream cheese

1 teaspoon ground turmeric

salt and ground white pepper

freshly chopped chives, to garnish

For the pickled red onion garnish

½ small red onion, very thinly sliced

2 tablespoons red wine vinegar

Start by preparing the pickled red onion garnish. Simply place the thinly sliced red onion in a small bowl and pour over the red wine vinegar. Set aside.

Preheat the oven to 200°C/180°C fan/400°F/gas mark 6.

Remove the sausages from their packaging and slice each one in half diagonally. This maximises their surface area. More surface area = more caramelisation = more flavour!

Melt the lard or ghee in a large non-stick frying pan over a high heat. Add the sausage pieces, cut-side down first. Cook for 1–2 minutes, then flip them over and brown on all sides for 1–2 minutes. Use tongs to remove the sausages from the pan and set them aside on a plate, leaving all the fat in the pan. Do not worry about whether they are cooked through – they will go in the oven later. This step is just to maximise flavour by caramelising the outside of the sausages.

Reduce the heat to low and add the garlic. Cook for 1–2 minutes until softened, then add the spinach. Cook until the spinach has completely wilted, stirring continuously. You may need to add the spinach in 2 batches if there isn't enough space in the pan at first.

Whisk together the double cream, soured cream and cream cheese in a bowl. Add the turmeric to the pan of spinach, then pour in the cream mixture. Stir well to combine and increase the heat to medium–high, cooking for 2 minutes to allow the cream to warm through and reduce a little. Season with salt and ground white pepper. Transfer the whole lot into a medium-sized, deep, ovenproof dish. Add the sausages and bake, uncovered, for 30 minutes. Serve scattered with freshly chopped chives and the all-important drained pickled red onion.

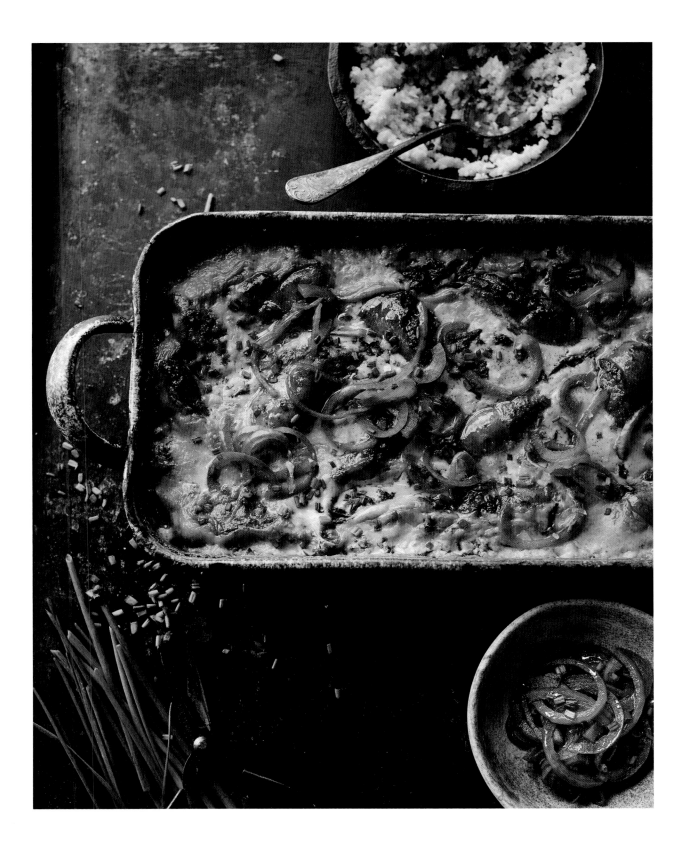

Bacon & Caramelised Onion Risotto

This delicious 'risotto' is packed with the flavour of salty, smoky bacon lardons, which is balanced beautifully by the sweet caramelised onions. I use konjac (shirataki) 'rice' here – please see my notes on page 7 for tips on how to prepare this so you can enjoy it at its best. This risotto makes an easy, satisfying dinner, and takes no time at all to throw together. *Pictured on pages 104 and 105.*

2 SERVINGS **10m** PREP TIME **25m** COOK TIME

CALORIES 717 | CARBOHYDRATES 6.4G | PROTEIN 30G | FAT 61G

400g (14oz) konjac (shirataki) 'rice'

1 tablespoon unsalted butter

250g (9oz) smoked bacon lardons

3 garlic cloves, finely chopped

½ large onion, finely chopped

60g (2¼oz) soured cream

50ml (2fl oz) double cream

20g (¾oz) Parmesan cheese, finely grated

freshly ground black pepper

small handful of fresh flat-leaf parsley leaves, finely chopped, to garnish

Prepare the konjac 'rice' according to the instructions on page 7.

Meanwhile, melt the butter in a large non-stick frying pan or wok over a medium heat. Add the bacon lardons and cook for 6–7 minutes. The bacon will start to release all its juices and begin to simmer. Add the garlic and continue to cook for a further 2–3 minutes until the garlic has softened and the bacon is cooked through and is just starting to caramelise and crisp.

Use a slotted spoon to remove the bacon and garlic mixture from the pan and set aside on a plate.

Add the onion to the same pan (which should still have plenty of fat in it) and reduce the heat to medium–low. Cook until the onion completely breaks down and starts to darken and caramelise – this can take up to 15 minutes. Be patient – the results are worth the wait, because the onion becomes sweet when cooked over a low heat like this, which will balance the saltiness of the bacon beautifully.

Return the bacon to the pan, along with the drained konjac 'rice'. Add the soured cream, double cream and grated Parmesan. Increase the heat to medium for 1–2 minutes, stirring well to combine and warm the whole lot through.

Serve scattered with chopped parsley for a fresh garnish. It is unlikely you will need any salt seasoning due to the salty smoked bacon, but a crack of freshly ground black pepper is always ideal. Simple and delicious!

Cabanossi Bolognese

I wanted to add a little something special to a Bolognese, so here I enhanced the mixture with some finely chopped cabanossi (see Tip), which adds a subtle smoky element to an otherwise ordinary midweek meal. This dish is excellent with a splash of hot sauce (my husband wanted me to add that), but I love it with a simple scattering of grated Parmesan and the all-important fresh basil. It's almost too easy... *Pictured on page 105.*

4 SERVINGS   **15m** PREP TIME   **50m** COOK TIME

CALORIES 535 | CARBOHYDRATES 8.1G | PROTEIN 30G | FAT 42G

400g (14oz) can chopped tomatoes

200ml (7fl oz) water

2 tablespoons double-concentrate tomato purée

2 tablespoons unsalted butter

2 garlic cloves, finely chopped

200g (7oz) mushrooms, finely chopped

2 teaspoons dried oregano

250g (9oz) minced beef, 20 per cent fat

200g (7oz) cabanossi, diced very small

9–10 fresh basil leaves, thinly sliced

4 tablespoons finely grated Parmesan cheese

salt flakes and freshly ground black pepper

Place the chopped tomatoes in a food processor along with the water and the tomato purée. Blitz well until smooth, then set aside.

Melt the butter in a large non-stick frying pan or wok over a medium heat. Add the garlic and cook for 1–2 minutes until softened. Add the mushrooms and oregano and continue to cook for 5–6 minutes until the mushrooms have completely softened and are beginning to caramelise. Add the minced beef and increase the heat to high. Cook, breaking up the mince with your spoon, for 8–10 minutes until the mince has browned.

Add the blitzed tomato mixture to the pan and reduce the heat to medium. Cook for about 20 minutes, stirring occasionally. Stir in the diced cabanossi and most of the sliced basil leaves (setting some aside to garnish). Stir well to combine and leave to cook, still over a medium heat, for 5–10 minutes until you have a thick, chunky Bolognese texture.

Serve over your choice of base, such as courgette noodles or konjac (shirataki) 'pasta', and season with salt flakes (if needed) and plenty of freshly ground black pepper. Scatter over the grated Parmesan and finish with the remaining fresh basil to garnish.

*

Cabanossi is a thin, cured pork sausage with a lovely smoked flavour. It is also called kabanas or kabana and can be found in the deli meat aisle.

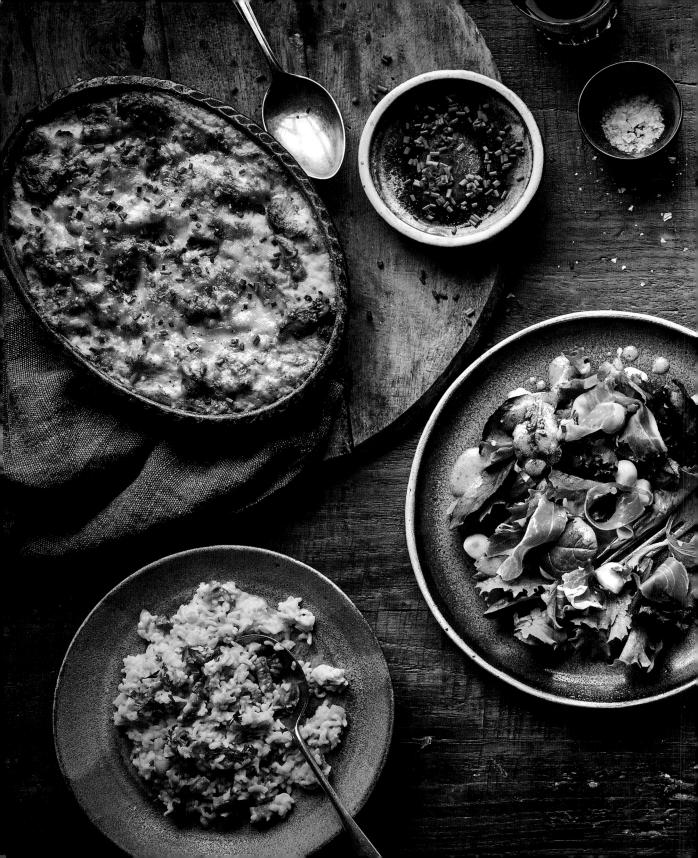

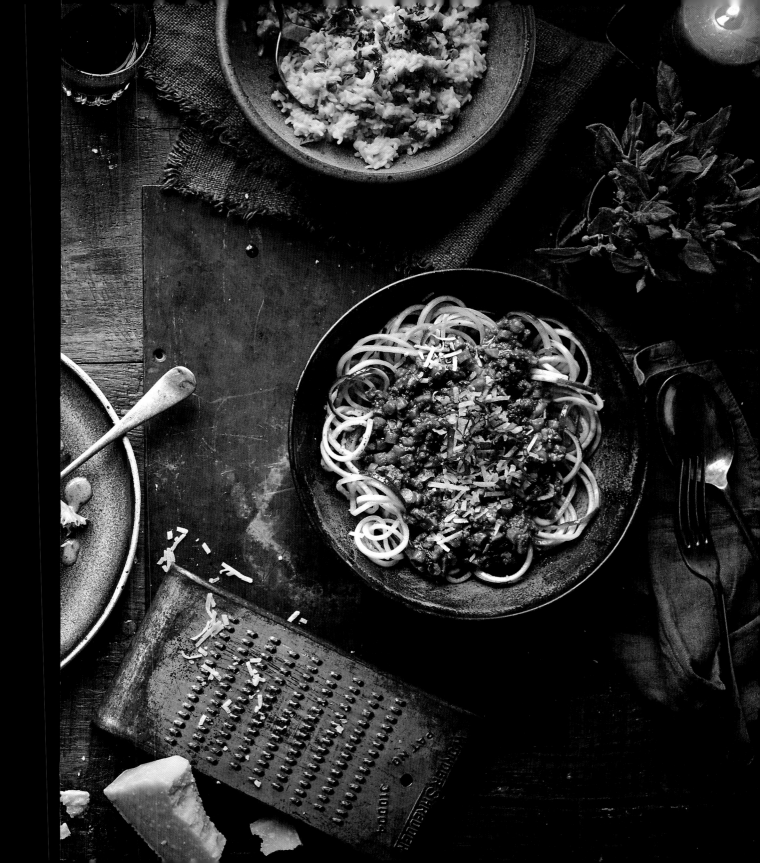

Sausage & Cauliflower Bake

This recipe is so simple and so tasty. The whole family (especially the kids) will love all the comforting flavours. It goes really well with a lovely, fresh salad on the side to cut through the richness. Be sure to use Gruyère cheese, as I am not sure any other cheese would pack the same punch. This is a firm favourite in our home, and we simply love it! *Pictured on page 104.*

4 SERVINGS | **15m** PREP TIME | **50m** COOK TIME

CALORIES 493 | CARBOHYDRATES 7G | PROTEIN 30G | FAT 38G

8 gluten-free pork sausages

650g (1lb 7oz) cauliflower florets

85g (3oz) full-fat cream cheese

55g (2oz) Gruyère cheese, finely grated

salt flakes, salt, ground white pepper and freshly ground black pepper

freshly chopped chives, to garnish

Preheat the oven to 220°C/200°C fan/425°F/gas mark 7.

Place the sausages in a greased ovenproof dish and bake for 20–25 minutes until golden and crispy. Remove the dish from the oven and set the sausages aside to cool, but leave the oven on.

Meanwhile, bring a large saucepan of salted water to the boil and add the cauliflower florets. Cook for 15–20 minutes until very soft. Drain well in a colander and leave to steam off for a few minutes to remove any excess wateriness.

Return the cauliflower to the saucepan you cooked it in (wipe the pan dry if needed) and add the cream cheese. Use a potato masher to mash the mixture, then place the saucepan over a very low heat so that any additional moisture can evaporate, ensuring you are not left with a watery bake. Once you are happy, season generously with salt and ground white pepper.

Chop the cooked, cooled sausages into bite-sized pieces and add to the mashed cauliflower. If there is any rendered fat from the sausages, add this, too. (Never waste rendered fat or resting juices: this is flavour!) Stir gently to combine, then tip the whole lot into a medium-sized ovenproof dish.

Scatter over the grated Gruyère and bake for 15–20 minutes until the cheese is bubbling. If you like, you can crank up the oven temperature to max for the last 3–4 minutes to get the cheese to really 'gratin' and crisp up.

Season with salt flakes and freshly ground black pepper, and garnish with plenty of freshly chopped chives. Serve with your favourite salad or buttered greens on the side.

Egg-fried 'Rice'

With a little effort, konjac (shirataki) products can be a keto game-changer. This simple egg-fried 'rice' has all the delicious flavours you would expect, with dried chilli flakes for an additional kick and a drizzle of the all-important toasted sesame oil just before serving. This delicious dish will satisfy two people as a main meal (as the macros show) or four as a side option. *Pictured on page 83.*

2 SERVINGS   **15m** PREP TIME   **10m** COOK TIME

CALORIES 317 | CARBOHYDRATES 3.4G | PROTEIN 16G | FAT 25G

400g (14oz) konjac (shirataki) 'rice'

20g (¾oz) unsalted butter

2 garlic cloves, finely chopped

8 spring onions, white parts thickly sliced, green parts thinly sliced

4 large eggs, whisked

1 tablespoon tamari (gluten-free soy sauce)

1 teaspoon dried chilli flakes

1 tablespoon toasted sesame oil

small handful of fresh coriander leaves, finely chopped (optional)

Prepare the konjac 'rice' according to the instructions on page 7.

Meanwhile, melt the butter in a large non-stick frying pan or wok over a low heat. Add the garlic and cook for 1–2 minutes until softened. Add the white spring onion slices and increase the heat to medium. Cook for 1 minute, stirring continuously so that the garlic doesn't burn. You will notice the spring onions turn bright green and will start to soften.

Tip in the drained konjac 'rice', along with the whisked eggs. Increase the heat to medium–high and cook for 2–3 minutes, stirring continuously to ensure the eggs cook properly. Add the tamari and dried chilli flakes, stirring well for a minute or two to combine and warm all the elements through.

Just before serving, drizzle over the toasted sesame oil and garnish with the green spring onion slices and chopped coriander (if using). Delicious!

Mini Rosemary Rolls

These mini bread rolls are a little like dumplings, and I love to bake them in an attractive cast-iron pan and then serve straight from it, tear-and-share-style. You can play around with different herbs, but I think I rocked these using rosemary. They are lovely with a spread of butter and will go brilliantly with a lamb dish, like the Lamb Shanks with Herby Tomato 'Gravy' (page 91). Macros shown are per roll, and this recipe makes a baker's dozen.

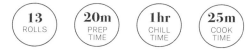

13 ROLLS | **20m** PREP TIME | **1hr** CHILL TIME | **25m** COOK TIME

CALORIES 107 | CARBOHYDRATES 1.5G | PROTEIN 5G | FAT 8.7G

100g (3½oz) grated mozzarella cheese

2 large eggs

80g (2¾oz) full-fat cream cheese

115g (4oz) almond flour

½ teaspoon salt

1 teaspoon garlic powder

1½ teaspoons baking powder

2–3 fresh rosemary sprigs, needles picked and finely chopped

½ teaspoon psyllium husk powder

Place the grated mozzarella in a shallow, microwave-safe bowl and microwave on high for 60–90 seconds until melted. Set aside.

Blitz the eggs and cream cheese in a food processor until smooth. The melted mozzarella will be cool enough by now to add to the eggs, so add it to the food processor and blitz again until smooth.

In a bowl, mix together the almond flour, salt, garlic powder, baking powder and chopped rosemary. Add this mixture to the food processor and blitz until well combined. Finally, add the psyllium husk powder and blitz one last time. Transfer the mixture to a clean bowl and place in the refrigerator, covered, for 1 hour to firm up.

Preheat the oven to 200°C/180°C fan/400°F/gas mark 6.

Divide the mixture into 13 small portions (approximately 30g/1oz each) and roll each one lightly into a ball. Place the balls into a medium-sized baking tin or a 20cm (8in) cast-iron pan lined with baking paper, leaving a little space between each one as they will puff up and rise.

Bake for 5 minutes, then reduce the oven temperature to 170°C/150°C fan/340°F/gas mark 3½ and bake for an additional 15 minutes. Turn off the oven, leaving the rolls inside for 5 minutes more to finish cooking gently in the residual heat.

Serve immediately (and please warn your guests about the hot pan if you're serving straight from the pan like me!).

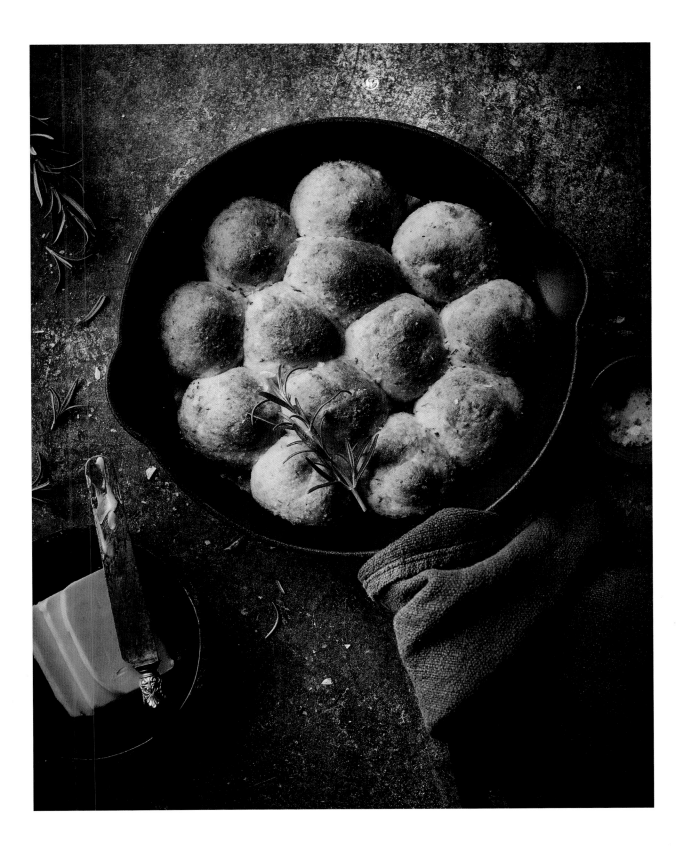

Cumin Flatbreads

These flatbreads are flavoured with partially crushed cumin seeds, meaning they make an excellent accompaniment to your Friday night curry! You can make plain flatbreads by simply omitting the cumin seeds, but I want to encourage you to play around, adding your choice of dried herbs or crushed spices to enhance the flavour and complement your meal! Partially crushing whole seeds will release flavour, as well as offering a little texture, so do avoid using ground spice powders with this one. *Pictured on page 89.*

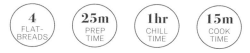

4 FLAT-BREADS | 25m PREP TIME | 1hr CHILL TIME | 15m COOK TIME

CALORIES 299 | CARBOHYDRATES 3.7G | PROTEIN 15G | FAT 24G

100g (3½oz) almond flour

¼ teaspoon salt

1 teaspoon garlic powder

½ tablespoon cumin seeds

100g (3½oz) grated mozzarella cheese

60g (2¼oz) full-fat plain yogurt

1 large egg, whisked

2 tablespoons ghee

1 garlic clove, crushed with a garlic press

salt flakes

small handful of fresh coriander leaves, finely chopped

In a bowl, mix together the almond flour, salt and garlic powder. Use a pestle and mortar to lightly crush the cumin seeds, then stir these into the mixture, too. Tip the whole lot into a food processor.

Place the grated mozzarella in a wide-bottomed, microwave-safe bowl and microwave on high for 60–90 seconds until the cheese melts. Carefully remove the bowl from the microwave and stir in the yogurt. Mix well to combine, then tip the mixture into the food processor containing the dry ingredients. Blitz the mixture well to combine. You may need to stop every now and then to pull the stringy mozzarella away from the blades, as it tends to wrap around them. Add the whisked egg and continue to mix until the mixture comes together to form a sticky dough. Transfer to a shallow bowl and leave in the refrigerator, covered, for 1 hour to firm up.

Preheat the oven to 180°C/160°C fan/350°F/gas mark 4 and line a baking tray with baking paper or a silicone mat.

Divide the chilled dough into 4 equally sized portions and place them on the prepared tray. Lay a sheet of baking paper on top and use your hands to flatten the mounds into discs measuring approximately 12cm (4½in) in diameter. They should be about 8mm (⅜in) thick. Peel away the top sheet of baking paper and bake the flatbreads for 5 minutes. Reduce the oven temperature to 160°C/140°C fan/325°F/gas mark 3 and bake for a further 10 minutes.

Meanwhile, melt the ghee in a small frying pan over a low heat and add the crushed garlic. Gently heat through for 1–2 minutes. Just before serving the flatbreads, brush them with the garlic ghee and scatter with salt flakes and finely chopped coriander.

Cheesy Celeriac Mash

This delicious low-carb mash is extra special because it boasts a cheesy creaminess, making it ideal to mop up all those lovely keto gravies and sauces. It is extraordinarily rich, but very versatile. If you are serving it alongside lamb, try stirring through a little finely chopped fresh rosemary; for chicken, try adding some thyme; or for fish, experiment with tarragon or dill. It's also perfectly tasty just as it is. *Pictured on page 90.*

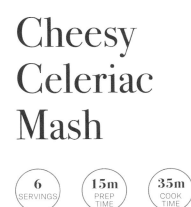

6 SERVINGS | **15m** PREP TIME | **35m** COOK TIME

CALORIES 264 | CARBOHYDRATES 3.3G | PROTEIN 7.4G | FAT 24G

750g (1lb 10oz) celeriac, peeled and diced into 2cm (¾in) pieces (trimmed weight)

160ml (5½fl oz) double cream

130g (4¾oz) extra-mature full-fat Cheddar cheese, grated

1 tablespoon unsalted butter

salt flakes, salt, ground white pepper and freshly ground black pepper

Bring a large saucepan of salted water to the boil and add the celeriac. Cook until the pieces have completely softened: they should slide off a fork if pierced. Drain well in a colander and leave for a few minutes to steam off. This will prevent a watery mash.

Return the celeriac to the saucepan you cooked it in (wipe the pan dry if needed) and use a potato masher to mash well, adding the cream and Cheddar halfway through. Season the mixture with salt and ground white pepper.

For an extra creamy mash, transfer the mixture to a food processor and blitz until completely smooth. Keep warm and stir through the butter for extra richness just before serving. Season with salt flakes and freshly ground black pepper. Delicious!

Cheesy 'Gnocchi'

I am delighted with these little pillows of cheesy 'gnocchi'! This is a basic, undressed recipe, so serve it with your favourite sauce, or simply drizzle with olive oil and scatter over fresh thyme leaves and lemon zest (as pictured) and enjoy it as a side option to your fish or chicken. Admittedly, there is quite a bit of prep time involved, but this is largely due to the need to chill the dough. This recipe could easily serve 3–4 people as a side dish option, as it is very rich and filling, but the macros are based on 2 cheese-lovers.

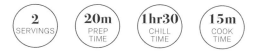

2 SERVINGS | **20m** PREP TIME | **1hr30** CHILL TIME | **15m** COOK TIME

CALORIES 537 | CARBOHYDRATES 4G | PROTEIN 27G | FAT 46G

180g (6½oz) grated mozzarella cheese

40g (1½oz) full-fat cream cheese (see Tip)

1 large egg, plus 1 large yolk

¼ teaspoon baking powder

¼ teaspoon garlic powder

olive oil, for greasing

3 tablespoons unsalted butter

salt

*

You can make the gnocchi (up to the point before rolling them with oiled hands) ahead of time, keeping the little balls of 'dough' covered in the refrigerator for up to 3 days.

Place the mozzarella in a wide-bottomed, microwave-safe bowl and microwave on high for 60–90 seconds until melted. Carefully pour the melted cheese into a food processor. Add the cream cheese and blitz well to combine. In a small jug or bowl, whisk together the egg and egg yolk and season with a little salt. Sift in the baking powder and add the garlic powder, whisking very well. Add to the food processor and blitz to combine. Tip the mixture out on to a tray lined with baking paper and spread it out a little. Cover with a second sheet of baking paper and chill for at least 1 hour until completely cold and firm.

Take little portions of dough (no more than 12g/¼oz each) and place them on 2 more trays lined with baking paper. Chill for another 30 minutes to firm up still further.

Roll 1 tray of gnocchi at a time, while the other tray remains in the refrigerator. Use clean, cold hands to roll each portion into a little ball, then pour a little olive oil into the palm of your hand and roll each piece into a smooth little log shape.

To cook, bring a large saucepan of salted water to a simmer over a medium heat. Tip in half the gnocchi and watch as they rise to the surface and puff up. Once they are floating, leave them to cook for a further 2 minutes. Remove the gnocchi with a slotted spoon and set aside on a clean plate or tray, then repeat with the second batch.

To finish, melt half the butter in a large non-stick frying pan over a medium–high heat. Once it's foaming, add half the gnocchi and gently fry for 1–2 minutes until they are golden on all sides. Remove and set aside to keep warm while you repeat the process with the remaining butter and gnocchi. Serve with your chosen accompaniments.

*

Tip out the excess liquid
from the container of cream
cheese to avoid a wet dough
that may be tricky to
work with.

Pickled Mushrooms
with Avocado & Feta Salad

This is a zingy side dish which would be perfect alongside a fatty cut of meat, as the acidity of the pickled mushrooms and red onion will cut through any richness. The flavour is quite strong, so I add feta and avocado to offer a milder flavour element and a creamy texture to the salad. The pickled onions don't actually need to be pickled overnight like the mushrooms – they only really need about 45 minutes, but you may as well do them at the same time. *Pictured on page 75.*

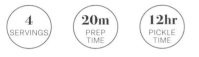

4 SERVINGS | **20m** PREP TIME | **12hr** PICKLE TIME

CALORIES 184 | CARBOHYDRATES 2G | PROTEIN 3.7G | FAT 17G

For the pickled mushrooms

250g (9oz) button mushrooms, halved if large

apple cider vinegar, for pickling

2 fresh dill sprigs

2 fresh flat-leaf parsley sprigs

1 teaspoon whole black peppercorns

2 garlic cloves, peeled

For the pickled red onion

¼ red onion, very thinly sliced

1 tablespoon red wine vinegar

For the salad

4 handfuls of mixed salad leaves

squeeze of fresh lemon juice

1 large avocado, peeled, stoned and diced

50g (1¾oz) full-fat feta cheese, crumbled

2 tablespoons olive oil

ground white pepper and freshly ground black pepper

fresh dill sprigs, to garnish

To make the pickled mushrooms, place the mushrooms into a wide, shallow bowl or jar and cover with equal amounts of cold water and apple cider vinegar. The mushrooms need to be completely submerged in the mixture, so be mindful of the size of your vessel so that you do not waste an unnecessarily large amount of vinegar. Add the dill, parsley and black peppercorns. Smash the peeled garlic cloves with the back of a knife and add those too. Cover and leave in the refrigerator overnight, or for at least 12 hours.

For the pickled red onion, place the red onion in a small, shallow bowl and pour over the red wine vinegar. Cover and leave in the refrigerator (see above). Give both the mushrooms and red onion a quick stir every so often to ensure even pickling.

When you're ready to assemble the salad, drain the mushrooms very well (discarding all the pickling elements). Be sure to check for any peppercorns in among the mushrooms (no one wants to bite into one of those!). Drain the pickled red onion and set aside.

Pat the mushrooms dry with paper towels and place them in a salad bowl. Add the salad leaves and toss together. Squeeze a little lemon juice over the avocado to prevent browning, then lightly season with ground white pepper and add it to the salad, along with the crumbled feta.

Finish the salad with the olive oil and top with the drained pickled red onion. Season with a generous crack of black pepper to balance the saltiness of the feta.

Scatter over a few sprigs of fresh dill for a beautiful finish.

Radish & Green Bean Salad

This interesting and pretty salad uses two low-carb vegetables that are often overlooked: radishes and green beans. The wholegrain mustard in the dressing is an essential acidic element that brings all the components together. The salad itself can be prepared ahead of time, but (as with all salads) the dressing should be added just before serving. It will serve 4–6 people as a side option, but the macros are calculated to serve 6, making it a perfect side salad for your next *braai* (barbecue) spread. *Pictured on page 79.*

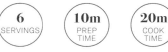

6 SERVINGS | **10m** PREP TIME | **20m** COOK TIME

CALORIES 138 | CARBOHYDRATES 2.9G | PROTEIN 4.9G | FAT 11G

300g (10½oz) fine green beans, trimmed (trimmed weight)

200g (7oz) radishes, halved

1 teaspoon olive oil, plus 1 tablespoon to finish

100g (3½oz) fresh mozzarella cheese, drained and torn into small pieces

2 generous handfuls of salad leaves (see Tip)

salt

For the dressing

2 tablespoons olive oil

2 tablespoons wholegrain mustard

1 teaspoon apple cider vinegar

salt and freshly ground black pepper

*

I like using lamb's lettuce in this salad, but any salad leaves will do.

Preheat the oven to 200°C/180°C fan/400°F/gas mark 6.

Bring a large saucepan of salted water to the boil. Add the green beans and cook for about 4 minutes until tender but still with a little bite, then drain and plunge into a bowl of iced water to prevent further cooking. Once the beans have cooled completely, drain well and set aside.

In a bowl, toss the halved radishes in the 1 teaspoon of olive oil and season with a little salt. Spread out on a baking tray and roast for about 10 minutes, just long enough to remove their raw flavour. Remove and set aside to cool.

Make a quick dressing by whisking together the olive oil, mustard and cider vinegar. Season with salt and freshly ground black pepper. Toss the cooled green beans and radishes in a bowl with the mozzarella pieces and dressing.

Arrange the salad leaves in a salad bowl and scatter the green-bean-and-radish mixture over the top. Drizzle with the remaining 1 tablespoon of olive oil and serve.

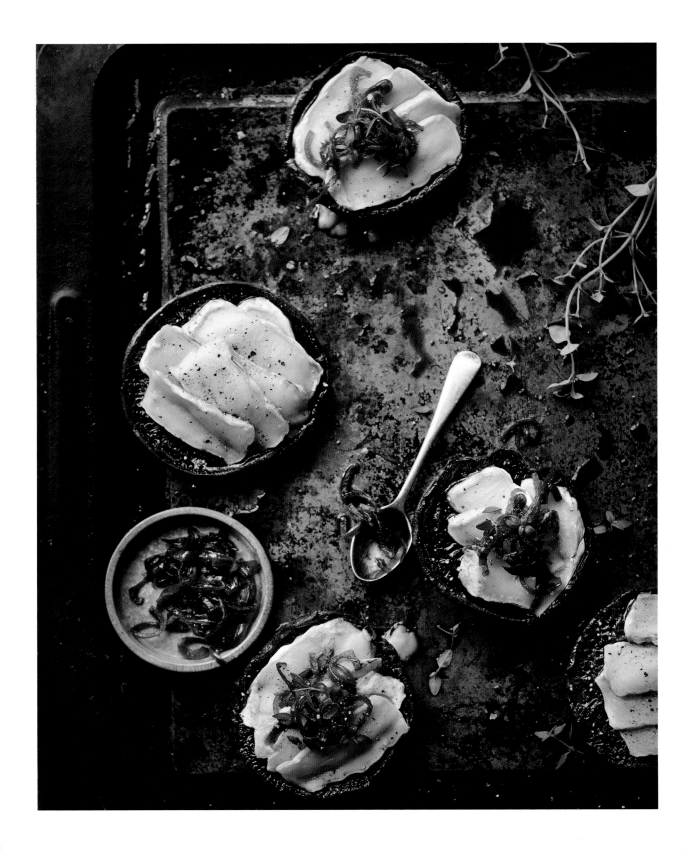

Cheesy Mushrooms

with Quick Red Onion 'Chutney'

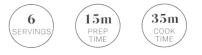

6 SERVINGS | **15m** PREP TIME | **35m** COOK TIME

The jammy sweetness of this slowly cooked onion 'chutney' balances the flavourful Camembert just perfectly as it melts into the giant umami-packed portobello mushrooms. At only 1.9g carbs per cheesy mushroom, you will probably want two – and there is no judgement here if you do! If you love this as much as I do, consider serving these as a topping for your steak, or even your bun-less burger – you will never consider a bacon and Cheddar topping again!

CALORIES 162 | CARBOHYDRATES 1.9G | PROTEIN 9.5G | FAT 13G

2 teaspoons unsalted butter

1 red onion, very thinly sliced

1 tablespoon red wine vinegar

6 large portobello mushrooms – the biggest you can get

1 tablespoon olive oil

240g (8½oz) best-quality Camembert or Brie

salt flakes and freshly ground black pepper

2–3 fresh thyme sprigs, leaves picked, to garnish

truffle-infused olive oil, for drizzling (optional)

*

I love using Camembert or Brie in this recipe, but you could also try it with a creamy blue cheese for an even stronger flavour!

Melt the butter in a small saucepan over a medium heat and add the onion. Cook for 10–12 minutes until completely softened. Add the vinegar to the pan, which will do a good job deglazing while adding a beautiful sweetness. Reduce the heat to low and continue to cook for about 15 minutes until the onion has softened still further and all the vinegar has evaporated. Set aside to keep warm.

Preheat the oven to 200°C/180°C fan/400°F/gas mark 6.

Gently remove the stalks from the mushrooms. (There is no need to discard the stalks – simply find another use for them, perhaps in another recipe that calls for chopped mushrooms.) Use a pastry brush to lightly brush the smooth side of each mushroom with olive oil, then place the mushrooms, gills facing down, on a roasting tray. Bake for 3 minutes, then remove the tray from the oven and turn the mushrooms over so the gills are facing up. (This initial 'upside down' bake helps prevent watery mushrooms, as it allows any released moisture to run off.)

Slice the Camembert or Brie into even-sized slices and place an equal amount on each mushroom. Return the tray to the oven for 4–5 minutes, or until the cheese melts a little. If the mushrooms still seem a little watery when you remove the tray, tip each one slightly to the side to allow the excess moisture to run off.

Serve the oozy mushrooms topped with the red onion 'chutney' and garnished with freshly picked thyme leaves. Finish with a small scatter of salt flakes and freshly ground black pepper. If you have any truffle-infused olive oil at hand, a drop or two on each mushroom after baking adds a sensational and luxuriously rich flavour!

Broccoli & Asparagus

with Lemon Dressing & Crackling Crumb

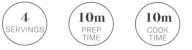

4 SERVINGS   **10m** PREP TIME   **10m** COOK TIME

While I simply love meat, I do pay a lot of attention to the accompanying side dishes. There is a multitude of things you can do with fresh vegetables to make them interesting and fun. These greens are drizzled with a beautiful dressing, and as they boast capers, lemon and tarragon, they will go beautifully alongside a fish dinner. *Pictured on page 51.*

CALORIES 186 | CARBOHYDRATES 3.9G | PROTEIN 7.8G | FAT 15G

230g (8¼oz) long-stem broccoli, trimmed (trimmed weight)

230g (8¼oz) asparagus, trimmed (trimmed weight)

100ml (3½fl oz) double cream

zest and juice of 1 lemon

1 garlic clove, crushed with a garlic press

1 teaspoon finely chopped fresh tarragon leaves

2 teaspoons small capers, drained

20g (¾oz) lean pork scratchings, crushed or blitzed in a mini food processor

salt flakes, salt and freshly ground black pepper

Bring a large saucepan of salted water to the boil. Add the broccoli and cook for 1–2 minutes, then add the asparagus and cook for a further 2 minutes. Remove the whole lot with tongs or a slotted spoon and place on to a tray lined with paper towels. Season with salt and set aside to keep warm.

Meanwhile, make the dressing by pouring the cream into a small saucepan and adding the lemon zest and juice (catch the pips!), along with the crushed garlic (see Tip). Gently warm the mixture over a low heat for 1–2 minutes before stirring through the chopped tarragon.

Place the broccoli and asparagus on a serving plate with the warm dressing spooned over the top, and scatter over the capers and crushed pork scratchings. Season with salt flakes and freshly ground black pepper and serve.

*

As the garlic in this dressing is almost raw, a garlic press is highly advised to achieve the best flavour and texture.

Baked Broccoli

with Tomato Garlic Relish

4 SERVINGS   **10m** PREP TIME   **40m** COOK TIME

I love cream-baked broccoli: it is such a simple dish, and one I make often. In this version, I top the rich, creamy bake with a quick relish made from chopped tomato and crushed garlic, which adds an additional flavour dimension. I have got into the habit of putting this fresh tomato garlic 'relish' over so many things... it's just lovely! *Pictured on page 99.*

CALORIES 394 | CARBOHYDRATES 6G | PROTEIN 5.7G | FAT 38G

350g (12oz) broccoli (approx. 1 head)

230ml (8fl oz) double cream

50g (1¾oz) soured cream

50g (1¾oz) full-fat cream cheese

1 teaspoon unsalted butter

1 garlic clove, finely chopped

salt flakes, salt, ground white pepper and freshly ground black pepper

For the tomato relish

1 tomato, finely chopped

1 garlic clove, crushed with a garlic press

1 teaspoon olive oil

Preheat the oven to 200°C/180°C fan/400°F/gas mark 6.

Trim the broccoli into evenly sized pieces. Do not discard the stems – they are delicious. Slice these into 2cm (¾in) chunks so that they cook through sufficiently.

Bring a large saucepan of salted water to the boil. Add the broccoli and cook for 4–5 minutes until tender. Drain in a colander and allow to steam off completely (this is important to avoid a watery bake). Transfer the cooked broccoli into a medium-sized ovenproof dish, spreading it out into a fairly even layer. Set aside.

In a bowl, whisk together the double cream, soured cream and cream cheese until there are no lumps. Season generously with salt and ground white pepper.

Melt the butter in a small saucepan over a low heat and gently cook the garlic for 1–2 minutes until softened. Pour the cream mixture into the pan and heat the mixture through for 2–3 minutes, allowing the cream to reduce and thicken a little. Pour the mixture into the dish over the cooked broccoli and bake for 25 minutes.

Meanwhile, make the relish. Place the chopped tomato in a small bowl and add the crushed garlic. The garlic is eaten raw, so using a garlic press is essential to achieve the best texture. Stir in the olive oil and season with salt flakes and freshly ground black pepper.

Once the broccoli bake is ready to serve, spoon over the fresh tomato relish and season the dish with salt flakes (if needed) and freshly ground black pepper.

Cream-baked Cabbage
with Truffle Drizzle

This is such an indulgent way to enjoy cabbage: the softened inner leaves of Savoy cabbage are baked in a seasoned cream, then finished with a few drops of truffle-infused olive oil, making it luxurious and heavenly! Given the overpowering flavour of truffle, only a small drizzle is needed. This recipe will serve 4–6 people as a side dish, so I've calculated the macros based on a 100g (3½oz) cooked serving, which is generous for such a rich side dish. Be sure to serve this alongside a simple steak or chicken to avoid any competing flavours.

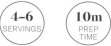

CALORIES 379 | CARBOHYDRATES 4.2G | PROTEIN 2.3G | FAT 39G

4–6 SERVINGS

10m PREP TIME

35m COOK TIME

1 tablespoon unsalted butter

2 garlic cloves, finely chopped

350g (12oz) Savoy cabbage, thinly sliced (see Tip)

350ml (12fl oz) double cream

salt flakes, salt, ground white pepper and freshly ground black pepper

truffle-infused olive oil, for drizzling

freshly chopped chives, to garnish

Preheat the oven to 200°C/180°C fan/400°F/gas mark 6.

Melt the butter in a large non-stick frying pan or wok over a medium heat. Once the butter is foaming, add the garlic and cook for 1 minute until softened. Tip in the thinly sliced cabbage and cook for 5–6 minutes, stirring continuously until the cabbage softens and completely wilts down.

Pour in the cream and season the mixture generously with salt and ground white pepper. Cook for 2–3 minutes to warm the cream through and reduce it a little.

Transfer the mixture into a medium-sized ovenproof dish, using a spatula to press it down to ensure the cabbage is submerged in the cream. Bake for 20–22 minutes until the surface is slightly caramelised.

Season with salt flakes and freshly ground black pepper and drizzle over a few drops of truffle-infused olive oil. Finish with freshly chopped chives and serve.

＊

You can use regular white cabbage if you prefer, but you may need to fry it for much longer to soften it sufficiently.

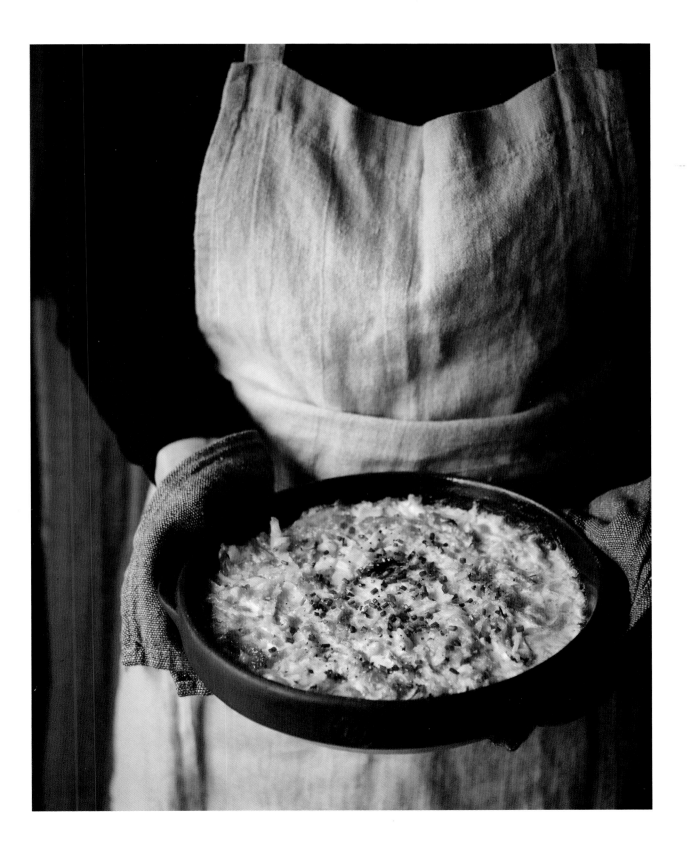

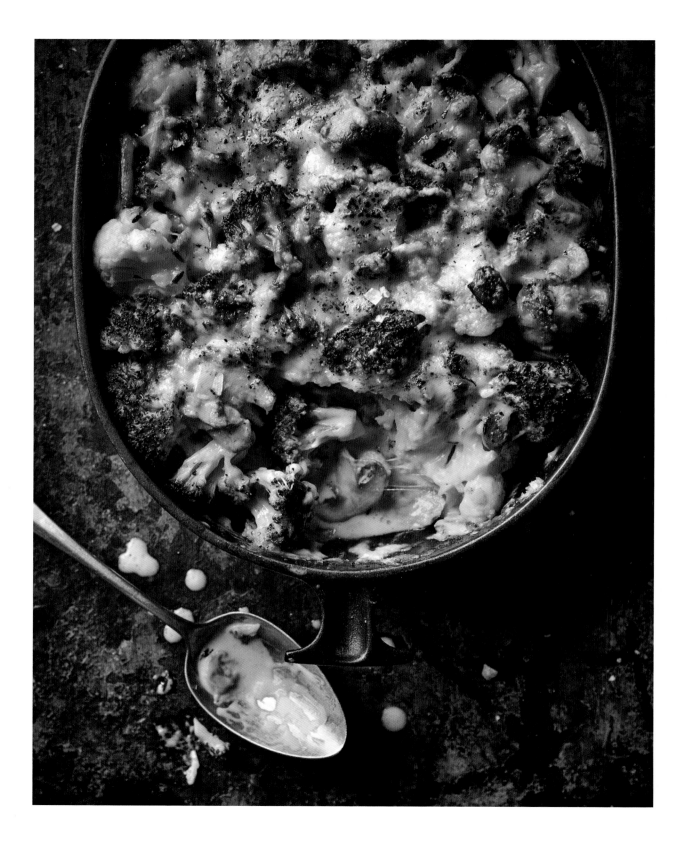

Decadent Vegetable Gruyère Bake

I am finishing off the vegetable side dish ideas with yet another creamy veg bake, because the flavour of baked cream is just so intoxicating – plus it's a great way to get your kids to eat more veg! Here I have included the beautiful flavour of Gruyère cheese. I've tried this bake with and without mushrooms, and both versions are fantastic, but the mushrooms bring a delicious umami flavour – and happen to be an excellent source of Vitamin D. Whip this out at your next Sunday roast – your family will love the rich decadence!

CALORIES 508 | CARBOHYDRATES 6.8G | PROTEIN 12G | FAT 48G

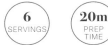
6 SERVINGS

20m PREP TIME

1hr COOK TIME

350g (12oz) cauliflower florets

300g (10½oz) broccoli florets

2 tablespoons unsalted butter

180g (6½oz) mushrooms, sliced

2–3 fresh thyme sprigs, leaves picked (see Tip)

3 garlic cloves, finely chopped

420ml (14¼fl oz) double cream

130g (4¾oz) Gruyère cheese, grated

pinch of paprika

salt flakes, salt, ground white pepper and freshly ground black pepper

*

If you don't have fresh thyme, you can use ¼ teaspoon of dried (dried herbs are more concentrated in flavour, so less is needed). Note, though, that dried herbs aren't great for garnishing dishes.

Preheat the oven to 200°C/180°C fan/400°F/gas mark 6.

Trim the cauliflower and broccoli florets into even-sized pieces, but keep them separate.

Bring a large saucepan of salted water to the boil and add the cauliflower. Boil rapidly for 3 minutes, then add the broccoli. Cook for a further 5–6 minutes until all the florets have softened but still retain their shape. Drain well in a colander and allow to steam off completely (this prevents a watery bake). Once this is done, transfer the vegetables into a medium–large ovenproof dish.

Meanwhile, melt 1½ tablespoons of the butter in a non-stick saucepan over a high heat (I just wipe the same saucepan I used to boil the vegetables and use that). Add the mushrooms and fry for 5–6 minutes until golden and caramelised. They will release some moisture, but continue to fry until this has evaporated. Add the remaining butter, along with the thyme leaves and garlic. Cook for 1 minute until the garlic softens, stirring continuously to prevent the garlic from burning.

Pour the cream into the pan and cook for 3–4 minutes to warm through and reduce a little. Stir in three-quarters of the grated Gruyère and season with the paprika, salt and ground white pepper. Pour the creamy mushroom mixture over the vegetables in the ovenproof dish. Mix well to combine, using a spatula to press the vegetables down to ensure they are mostly submerged in the cream. Scatter over the remaining Gruyère and bake for 25–30 minutes, cranking the oven temperature up to max for the last few minutes if needed to ensure the cheese gratins beautifully.

Just before serving, season with salt flakes (if needed) and freshly ground black pepper.

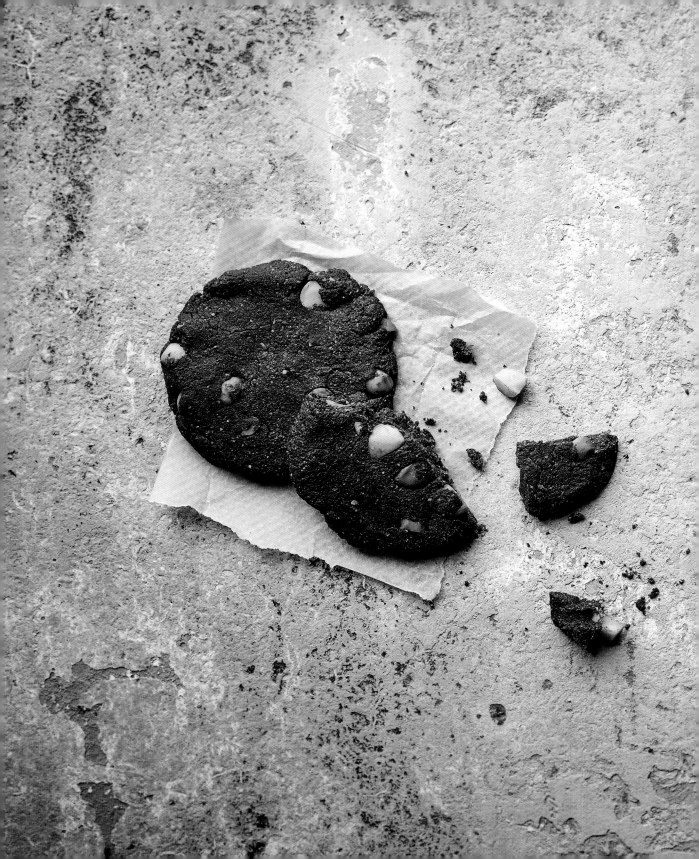

Something
Sweet

Lemon Cookie 'Sandwiches'

The first time I made a batch of these little lemon biscuits, we loved them, but I decided to add a little extra fun by turning them into 'sandwich' cookies with a lemon-flavoured cream cheese as the filling. If lemon is not to your liking, you can use vanilla instead, or try using cocoa powder for a chocolate option! Macros are per 'sandwich' cookie.

18 COOKIES | **30m** PREP TIME | **30m** CHILL TIME | **10m** COOK TIME

CALORIES 120 | CARBOHYDRATES 1.3G | PROTEIN 2.9G | FAT 11G

For the biscuits

1 large egg white

200g (7oz) almond flour

70g (2½oz) powdered erythritol, sifted

finely grated zest of 3 lemons

80g (2¾oz) unsalted butter, softened

3–4 drops of liquid stevia (optional)

For the cream cheese filling

100g (3½oz) full-fat cream cheese

1 teaspoon fresh lemon juice

½ tablespoon powdered erythritol, sifted

2 drops of liquid stevia (optional)

This dough is much easier to handle when chilled and needs to be handled gently. A palette knife is a great tool here for lifting and moving the delicate cookie dough.

Begin by making the biscuits. In a medium-sized bowl, use a hand mixer to whisk the egg white to meringue stage, then set aside.

In a large bowl, combine the almond flour, erythritol and lemon zest. Add the softened butter and use the hand mixer to mix until it resembles breadcrumbs. Add the whisked egg white and liquid stevia (if using) and mix until it comes together as a dough.

Tip the dough out on to a large sheet of baking paper and place a second sheet of baking paper on top. Use a rolling pin to roll it out to a thickness of about 5mm (¼in). Slide the dough on to a tray and chill for at least 30 minutes: this will make it easier to work with.

Preheat the oven to 180°C/160°C fan/350°F/gas mark 4 and line 2 baking trays with baking paper or silicone mats.

Peel off the top sheet of baking paper from the chilled dough and use a 5cm (2in) cookie cutter to cut out discs of dough. Gently lift them up (see Tip) and transfer to the prepared baking trays, leaving a little space between each biscuit. Do not discard the off-cuts: simply form the dough into a ball and roll it out again, repeating the cutting-out process so that no dough goes to waste. You should be able to press out about 36 biscuits if using every last bit of dough, so you'll probably need to bake the biscuits in 2 batches.

Bake for 7–8 minutes until golden brown, rotating the trays halfway through. Carefully transfer the biscuits to a wire rack to cool.

Whisk together the filling ingredients and top 18 of the cooled biscuits with a small amount of filling – about 5g (⅛oz) per biscuit. Use the remaining biscuits to form the top parts of the 'sandwiches' and very gently press down. Too cute!

*

I keep these in an airtight
container in the refrigerator –
surprisingly, they do not lose
their crispness.

Chocolate Mud Pie

This luxurious dessert is loosely based on a classic French silk pie. Depending on the temperature at which it is served, you can choose to have it super-silky (by removing it from the refrigerator 1 hour before enjoying) or more ganache-like (enjoyed straight from the refrigerator). Please be mindful that it contains raw eggs, so use the freshest eggs you can find and consume within 2 days of making (but I don't think that will be a problem at all!).

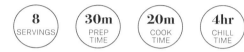

8 SERVINGS | **30m** PREP TIME | **20m** COOK TIME | **4hr** CHILL TIME

CALORIES 690 | CARBOHYDRATES 8.7G | PROTEIN 9.9G | FAT 68G

190g (6¾oz) dark chocolate (85 per cent cocoa), broken into small pieces, plus 10g (¼oz) grated, to decorate

120g (4¼oz) unsalted butter

450ml (16fl oz) double cream

60g (2¼oz) powdered erythritol, sifted

2 large eggs

1 tablespoon unsweetened cocoa powder

For the base

120g (4¼oz) almond flour

2 tablespoons powdered erythritol, sifted

1 tablespoon unsweetened cocoa powder

50g (1¾oz) unsalted butter

2–3 drops of liquid stevia (optional)

*

If 8.7g carbs seems a little high, simply slice the pie more thinly and stretch the decadence to 16 portions.

Begin by making the base. Preheat the oven to 200°C/180°C fan/400°F/gas mark 6 and grease a loose-bottomed 18cm (7in) tart tin.

In a bowl, mix together the almond flour, erythritol and cocoa powder. Gently melt the butter in a small saucepan over a low heat and add the liquid stevia (if using). Pour the melted butter into the almond flour mixture and stir well. Tip into the prepared tart tin and press down to form an even, compact layer on the base and up the sides of the tin. Bake for 12 minutes, then allow to cool completely in the tin on a wire rack. Once cooled, carefully remove the tart from the tin and place on a serving plate or cake stand.

Meanwhile, make the chocolate filling. Place the chocolate pieces and the butter in a small non-stick saucepan over a low heat and stir until melted. Set aside to cool to room temperature.

In a separate bowl, use a hand mixer to whip together the cream and erythritol until the mixture forms soft peaks. Transfer half of this sweetened whipped cream into a second bowl and set it aside for the chocolate cream topping.

Pour the melted chocolate into the first bowl of whipped cream and continue to mix with the hand mixer. Add the eggs, one at a time, mixing between each addition until the mixture is almost mousse-like. Immediately tip this mixture into the cooled tart case.

To make the chocolate cream topping, clean the whisks on your hand mixer, then whip the cocoa powder into the reserved bowl of sweetened cream until it forms stiff peaks. Gently spread this mixture on top of the mud pie and decorate with the grated chocolate. Leave to chill in the refrigerator for 3–4 hours before enjoying.

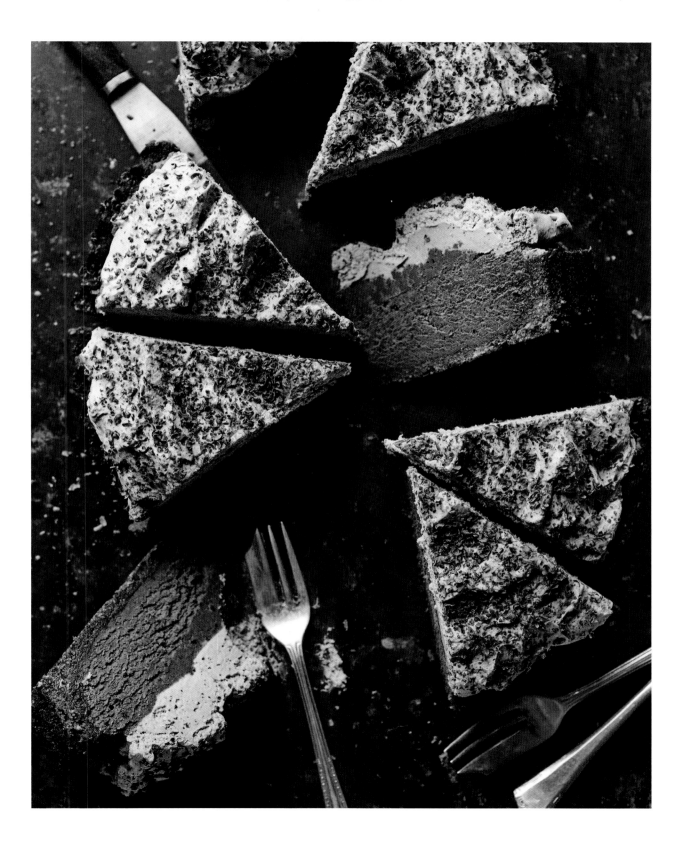

Turkish Delight

'White Chocolate' Mousse

6 SERVINGS | **20m** PREP TIME | **1hr** CHILL TIME

20g (¾oz) cocoa butter buttons (see Tip)

2–3 drops of liquid stevia (optional)

450ml (16fl oz) double cream

40g (1½oz) powdered erythritol, sifted

1 teaspoon rose water

pink food colouring (optional)

*

Cocoa butter buttons are also called 'raw cacao drops' or 'cacao chunks' and can be found in health food stores.

This easy white chocolate mousse uses only a few ingredients and features a distinct 'Turkish Delight' flavour due to the addition of rose water. It is a fragrant dessert that makes for a lovely dinner party treat. I've added a drop or two of pink food colouring, but that is optional.

CALORIES 381 | CARBOHYDRATES 1.8G | PROTEIN 1.1G | FAT 41G

Gently melt the cocoa butter buttons in a small saucepan over a low heat, then set aside to cool (to avoid a grainy mousse). Add a few drops of liquid stevia (if using).

In a large bowl, whip together the cream and erythritol until soft peaks form. Add the rose water and a few drops of pink food colouring (if using) and whip well again to combine. Drizzle the cooled melted cocoa butter into the mixture and whip one last time. The mixture will stiffen very quickly once the cocoa butter is added, so immediately spoon (or pipe) it into 6 dessert bowls. Cover each bowl and leave in the refrigerator for at least 1 hour to set before serving.

Little Raspberry Mousse Pots

6 SERVINGS | **20m** PREP TIME | **5m** COOK TIME | **2hr** CHILL TIME

2 tablespoons boiling water

1½ teaspoons gelatine powder

280g (10oz) fresh raspberries, plus extra to serve (optional)

1 teaspoon fresh lemon juice

230ml (8fl oz) double cream

3 tablespoons powdered erythritol, sifted

These fabulous little raspberry mousse pots will hit the spot when you are craving a high-fat sweet snack. Their luxuriously light and creamy texture is enhanced with a sharp sweetness from the raspberries, and they could not be easier to make.

CALORIES 206 | CARBOHYDRATES 3.2G | PROTEIN 2.2G | FAT 20G

Put the boiling water in a small ramekin and sprinkle over the gelatine powder. Leave for 3–4 minutes to completely dissolve. Set aside.

Place the raspberries and lemon juice in a mini food processor and blitz until smooth. Tip the purée into a small saucepan over a low heat and bring to a simmer. Add the gelatine mixture and stir well, cooking for 30–40 seconds more to incorporate. Set aside.

In a large bowl, use a hand mixer to whip together the cream and erythritol until semi-soft peaks form. Add the raspberry purée and mix to combine. Divide the bright pink mixture between 6 small dessert bowls and leave (covered) in the refrigerator to set for at least 2 hours. Enjoy topped with fresh raspberries, if you have any extra at hand.

*

Both these desserts can be
made up to 2 days ahead if
stored covered in the refrigerator.
(Just be sure to check the
date of the cream!)

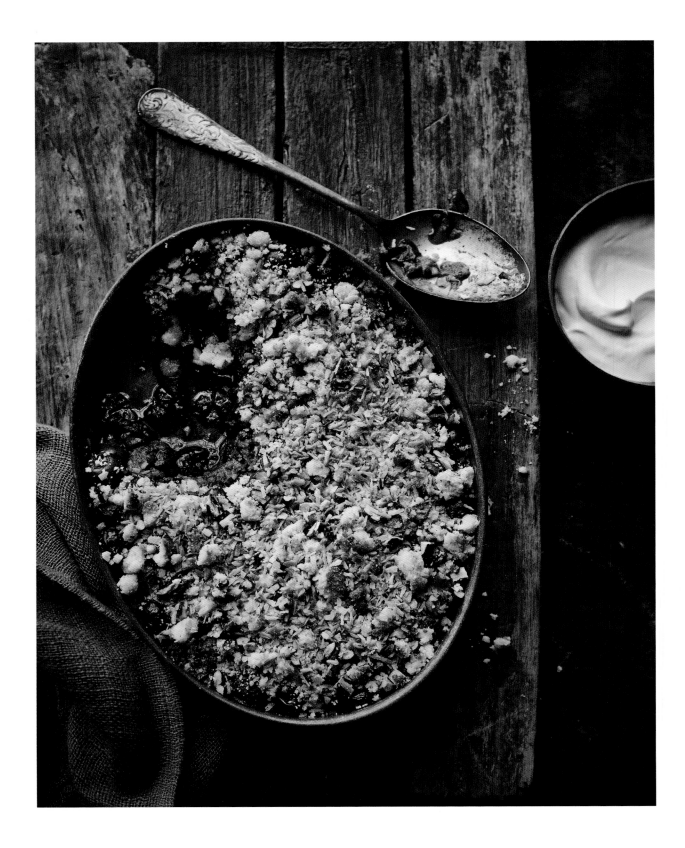

Cheat's Berry & Coconut Crumble

4–6 SERVINGS

15m PREP TIME

30m COOK TIME

This is a lovely, warm, keto-friendly dessert, where baked berries shine alongside a coconutty crumble. I cheated plenty here, baking some of the elements separately to ensure we achieve some texture in the crumble – and I bet your guests will not even know the difference! This dessert could serve 4–6 people, but the macros are based on a 120g (4¼oz) cooked serving per person. We love this with a little sweetened whipped cream (see Tip), which is optional but encouraged.

CALORIES 207 | CARBOHYDRATES 10G | PROTEIN 3.9G | FAT 15G

40g (1½oz) pecan nuts, finely chopped

15g (½oz) desiccated coconut

350g (12oz) fresh blueberries

150g (5½oz) fresh raspberries

1 teaspoon fresh lemon juice

2 tablespoons powdered erythritol, sifted

25g (1oz) almond flour

20g (¾oz) coconut flour

25g (1oz) unsalted butter, melted

*

Make a sweetened cream by using a hand mixer to whip 240ml (8¼fl oz) double cream with 3 tablespoons sifted erythritol until semi-soft peaks form.

Preheat the oven to 200°C/180°C fan/400°F/gas mark 6.

Spread out the chopped pecan nuts on a large baking tray. Toast in the oven for 4–5 minutes, then remove – but do not turn the oven off.

Meanwhile, heat a dry, non-stick frying pan over a medium heat and add the desiccated coconut. Toast until golden – and keep your eye on it as it can burn quickly. Set aside for use at the end.

Place the blueberries in a bowl and use the back of a fork to lightly crush and break the skins. Add the whole raspberries, along with the lemon juice and ½ tablespoon of the erythritol. Combine gently before tipping the whole lot into a 15 x 15cm (6 x 6in) ovenproof dish.

In another bowl, mix together the almond flour, coconut flour and the remaining erythritol. Add the toasted pecan nuts and pour over the melted butter. Combine well, then scatter evenly over the berry mixture. Bake for 10 minutes, then lay a sheet of foil (with a few holes poked into it) over the dish to prevent the top from browning too much. Bake for an additional 5 minutes, then turn off the oven, remove the foil and leave the crumble to continue browning in the residual heat (if needed) until you are satisfied with its golden topping.

Scatter over the toasted desiccated coconut and serve with sweetened whipped cream, if desired.

Blueberry Cheesecake

This delicious blueberry cheesecake will make 8 people incredibly happy! It doesn't have a dense cheesecake-like texture – in fact, it is light and almost mousse-like, which I simply love! Each generous slice comes in at only 5.2g carbs per serving, and you can get creative by decorating it with a scattering of fresh blueberries and a light dusting of powdered erythritol.

8 SERVINGS | **30m** PREP TIME | **25m** COOK TIME | **4hr** CHILL TIME

CALORIES 384 | CARBOHYDRATES 5.2G | PROTEIN 6.1G | FAT 37G

For the base

130g (4¾oz) almond flour

2 tablespoons powdered erythritol, sifted

45g (1½oz) unsalted butter

For the cheesecake filling

2 tablespoons boiling water

1½ teaspoons gelatine powder

150g (5½oz) fresh blueberries

200g (7oz) full-fat cream cheese

40g (1½oz) powdered erythritol, sifted

1 tablespoon fresh lemon juice

2–3 drops of liquid stevia (optional)

280ml (9½fl oz) double cream

Preheat the oven to 200°C/180°C fan/400°F/gas mark 6 and grease and line the base and sides of a deep, 20cm (8in) loose-bottomed/springform tin with baking paper.

To make the base, mix together the almond flour and erythritol in a bowl. Gently melt the butter in a small saucepan over a low heat, then pour it into the almond mixture. Stir well to combine, then tip the mixture into the prepared tin, pressing it down until you achieve a compact, even layer on the base of the tin.

Bake for 11–12 minutes, then set aside to cool.

To make the cheesecake filling, put the boiling water in a small ramekin and sprinkle over the gelatine powder. Leave for 3–4 minutes to completely dissolve. Set aside.

Place the blueberries in a small saucepan and add 1 tablespoon of water. Cook over a medium heat for 8–10 minutes, then use a potato masher to mash to a pulp. Stir in the gelatine mixture and mix well to thoroughly combine. Set aside to cool for 15 minutes.

Place the cream cheese, erythritol, lemon juice and liquid stevia (if using) in a bowl. Whisk together until smooth.

In a second, large bowl, whip the double cream until semi-soft peaks form. Add the cream cheese mixture, along with the blueberry mixture, and whip once more to fully combine. Immediately fill the springform tin with the mixture and smooth over the surface. Place in the refrigerator for at least 4 hours to set.

To serve, remove the cheesecake from the tin and peel away the baking paper from the sides before slicing and enjoying.

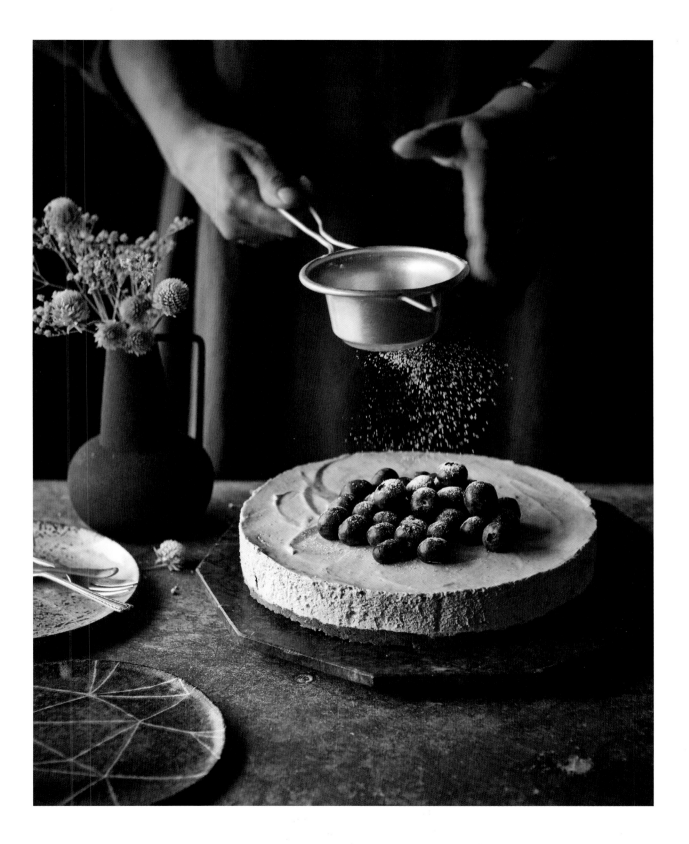

I had no idea what to call this: is it brittle? Is it fudge? Words like 'frittle' and 'budge' started floating around our home, but I settled on 'Buttery Brittle' before we started losing our minds. In a nutshell, this is a delicately crispy brittle that tastes like crystallised fudge! Break it into smaller pieces and get creative! My husband loves it as a topping on my Yogurt Pots (page 17) and Nut Butter Cream Shakes (page 138), but I love it most in the Crunchy Salted Caramel Lollies (opposite). Macros here are calculated on a 30g (1oz) serving.

CALORIES 152 | CARBOHYDRATES 2.7G | PROTEIN 3.4G | FAT 14G

Line a small baking tray with baking paper. Place the nuts on the tray. They should be in a single layer and relatively compact. Set aside.

Melt the butter in a small, non-stick saucepan over a medium heat, then stir in the erythritol. It may look like it's splitting, but it will come together and look glossy after about a minute. Add the vanilla, liquid stevia (if using) and 'maple' syrup. Increase the heat to high and stir continuously as it furiously bubbles away. It is tricky to give you a time indication, so I suggest you remove the pan from the heat after 2–3 minutes and allow the bubbling to stop so that you can see the colour. You want a dark, golden caramel. If you have a confectioner's thermometer, aim for 145°C (293°F), but it's OK to judge it by sight. If the caramel is undercooked, the mixture will be too brittle, but if it overcooks, it can become dark and burnt.

Once you are happy with the caramel, immediately drizzle it evenly over the laid-out nuts and leave to cool completely. It can take up to 2–3 hours to completely solidify. Store in a sealed container, breaking it up as necessary.

Mixed Nut Buttery Brittle

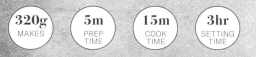

320g MAKES | **5m** PREP TIME | **15m** COOK TIME | **3hr** SETTING TIME

170g (6oz) roasted, salted mixed nuts, any larger ones chopped

60g (2¼oz) unsalted butter

100g (3½oz) powdered erythritol, sifted

1 teaspoon vanilla extract

1–2 drops of liquid stevia (optional)

2 tablespoons sugar-free 'maple' syrup

Crunchy Salted Caramel Lollies

6 LOLLIES | **15m** PREP TIME | **12hr** FREEZE TIME

250ml (9fl oz) double cream

100ml (3½fl oz) sugar-free 'salted caramel' syrup, plus extra to drizzle (optional)

120g (4¼oz) Mixed Nut Buttery Brittle (opposite), chopped

*

The macros here are based on 6 x 100ml (3½fl oz) moulds, with the lollies weighing approx. 80g (2¾oz) each.

I don't know why it took me so long to discover sugar-free 'salted caramel' syrup, but it's changed things here at our house quite significantly! With these tasty lollies, I snuck in some of my chopped Mixed Nut Buttery Brittle, which adds texture, crunch and heaps of flavour! If you are up for making them extra cute, brush the ends of the frozen lollies with a little syrup and roll them in any leftover finely chopped brittle. These lollies make it well worth investing in an inexpensive set of ice-lolly moulds!

CALORIES 294 | CARBOHYDRATES 2.4G | PROTEIN 2.9G | FAT 30G

In a large bowl, use a hand mixer to whip the double cream until stiff peaks form. Stir through the sugar-free 'salted caramel' syrup and the chopped brittle. Divide the mixture between 6 ice-lolly moulds. You could drizzle a little extra syrup into the moulds beforehand to achieve a pretty, 'marbled' effect.

Click the lid/stick into each mould and place in the freezer for 12 hours or overnight. Transfer the lollies to the refrigerator 30 minutes before eating, or simply run hot water on the outside of the moulds to make the lollies easier to slide out.

Nut Butter Cream Shakes

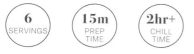

6 SERVINGS   **15m** PREP TIME   **2hr+** CHILL TIME

Creamy and very filling, these uncomplicated little shakes use store-bought, unsweetened almond nut butter and a handful of other ingredients. You could jazz them up by topping with whipped cream, a drizzle of sugar-free syrup and some chopped Mixed Nut Buttery Brittle (page 136) for utter decadence! The end yield will be enough for anything from 4–8 people, depending on your sweet tooth. They are incredibly rich, so I will leave it up to you to decide. As a guideline, the macros are calculated on 6 shakes, excluding any extras.

CALORIES 454 | CARBOHYDRATES 3.7G | PROTEIN 6.6G | FAT 46G

400ml (14fl oz) double cream

80g (2¾oz) powdered erythritol, sifted

300ml (10fl oz) unsweetened almond milk

120g (4¼oz) smooth unsweetened almond nut butter (see Tip), at room temperature

2–3 drops of liquid stevia (optional)

In a large bowl, use a hand mixer to whip together the cream and erythritol until semi-stiff peaks form.

In a separate bowl, use a hand blender to blitz together the almond milk, nut butter and liquid stevia (if using). Pour the almond butter mixture into the bowl of whipped cream and whip well to combine.

The shakes can be enjoyed as they are, but they are supremely better if served ice cold, in which case you should cover the mixture and place it in the refrigerator for at least 2 hours. If you are ambitious enough to own an ice-cream maker, you could partially churn the mixture (once chilled), giving it more of a 'milkshake' consistency.

*

You could use this method to make a cashew nut butter shake (6.1g carbs per serving), or, in the spirit of being 'dirty', a peanut butter version (4.7g carbs per serving).

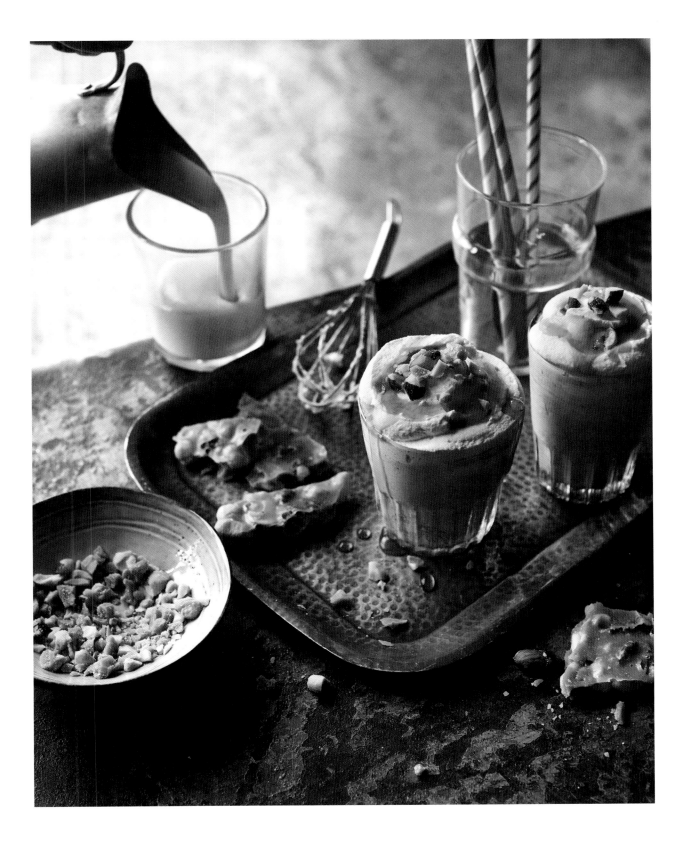

Chocolate & Macadamia Cookies

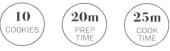

10 COOKIES   **20m** PREP TIME   **25m** COOK TIME

I love these delicious dark chocolate and macadamia cookies, which remind me of ones we enjoyed on our honeymoon all those years ago (life before keto!). I am thrilled that Mark and I can relive that memory with my low-carb version. These are dense and satisfying – and simply perfect dunked in a cup of Double Creamy Coffee (page 16)! *Pictured on page 124.*

CALORIES 289 | CARBOHYDRATES 5.5G | PROTEIN 7.5G | FAT 26G

80g (2¾oz) macadamia nut halves, roughly chopped

100g (3½oz) dark chocolate (85 per cent cocoa), broken into small pieces

30g (1oz) unsalted butter

1–2 drops of liquid stevia (optional)

200g (7oz) almond flour

100g (3½oz) powdered erythritol, sifted

2½ tablespoons unsweetened cocoa powder

1 large egg white

*

I always rotate my baking trays halfway through to ensure even cooking. If you do this, too, be sure to do so quickly to avoid the oven losing temperature while the door is open.

Preheat the oven to 180°C/160°C fan/350°F/gas mark 4 and line a large baking tray with baking paper (you may need 2 trays, depending on the size).

Spread out the chopped nuts on a separate small baking tray and roast for 8–9 minutes, shaking the tray halfway through. Remove from the oven and set aside, but leave the oven on.

Meanwhile, place the chocolate and butter in a small saucepan over a low heat and gently melt together. Add the liquid stevia (if using). Remove the pan from the heat and set aside to cool a little.

In a bowl, mix together the almond flour, erythritol and cocoa powder. In a separate bowl, whisk the egg white until it is foamy. Pour the melted chocolate mixture into the bowl containing the almond flour mixture. Stir quickly, then pour in the whisked egg white, along with the roasted nuts. It will quickly come together to form a dough.

Divide the dough into 10 equal portions and roll into balls before placing on the prepared baking tray(s). With clean hands, flatten and shape each ball to form a cookie, leaving a space between each cookie.

Bake for 9 minutes on the lowest rack in the oven, quickly rotating the tray halfway through (see Tip), then turn off the oven and leave the cookies to cook in the residual heat for an additional 6–7 minutes. This will ensure they cook through without burning.

Remove from the oven and leave to cool on the baking tray(s) for 10–15 minutes before using a spatula to gently slide each delicate cookie on to a wire rack. They will crisp up once they have cooled completely. Store in an airtight container. I keep mine in the refrigerator, but they are gone within a week!

Index

Index

References

McGee, Harold. *McGee on Food and Cooking: An Encyclopedia of Kitchen Science, History and Culture*, Hodder & Stoughton, 2004.

Noakes, Tim, Proudfoot, Jonno and Creed, Sally-Ann. *The Real Meal Revolution*, Robinson, 2015.

diabetes.org.uk/guide-to-diabetes/managing-your-diabetes/ketones-and-diabetes

healthline.com/nutrition/shirataki-noodles-101

healthline.com/nutrition/are-vegetable-and-seed-oilsbad#section5

healthline.com/health/oxidative-stress

healthline.com/health/gut-health

perfectketo.com/cacao-butter/

Recommended Reading

Chutkan, Robynne. *The Microbiome Solution*, Scribe UK, 2016.

Noakes, Tim, Proudfoot, Jonno and Creed, Sally-Ann. *The Real Meal Revolution*, Robinson, 2015.

Mosley, Michael. *The Clever Guts Diet*, Short Books, 2017.

Teicholz, Nina. *The Big Fat Surprise*, Scribe, 2015.

www.dietdoctor.com

www.zoeharcombe.com

www.thenoakesfoundation.org

UK/US Glossary

Ingredients
bicarbonate of soda – *baking soda*
biscuits – *cookies*
coriander – *cilantro*
celeriac – *celery root*
courgette – *zucchini*
dark chocolate – *bittersweet chocolate*
desiccated coconut – *dried shredded coconut*
dried chilli flakes – *dried hot red pepper flakes*
double cream – *heavy cream*
flaked almonds – *slivered almonds*
king prawns – *jumbo shrimp*
long-stem broccoli – *broccolini*
minced beef/pork – *ground beef/pork*
pepper (red/green) – *bell pepper/capsicum*
soured cream – *sour cream*
spring onions – *scallions*
stock – *broth*
swede – *rutabaga*
tomato purée – *tomato paste*

Equipment
baking paper – *parchment paper*
baking tray – *baking sheet*
clingfilm – *plastic wrap*
frying pan – *skillet*
loaf tin – *loaf pan*
muffin tray – *muffin pan*
piping bag – *pastry bag*
roasting tray – *roasting pan*
sieve – *fine mesh strainer*
tart tin – *tart pan*

Note on eggs
A large egg in the US is slightly different to a large egg in the UK. A UK medium egg is closer in size to a US large egg, and a UK large egg is closer in size to a US extra-large egg.

Acknowledgements

First and foremost, my thanks must go to Clare, my super-agent, who hooked me up with not one, but two book deals in less than twelve months. May there be many more, Clare!

To the wonderful people at Kyle: Judith, Jo, Florence, Jenny, Lisa and our designer Nicky – thank you for your hard work and dedication. To the lovely Tara, I could not ask for a better editor on my dream projects.

To our photographer, the (legendary) Maja Smend. I learn so much from you, thank you for being simply brilliant. Thank you also to Morag for the stunning props: it's those small details which make the visuals come alive, and I couldn't be more grateful! To Lisa and Phoebe, your hard work is deeply appreciated.

Creating a book is an enormous endeavour – and also happens to be a great way to practise some humility. Asking for help is something I struggle with, but the kindness and generosity I experienced from friends and strangers makes me want to do it more often!

To my wonderful friend, Gillian Harvey, who I 'met' through Professor Tim Noakes' Nutrition Network after completing an excellent course a few years back. How fortunate I am to be able to tap into the minds of this global network of nutritionists and medical professionals who are all passionately swimming against the current to promote the low-carb, high-(natural)-fat lifestyle and all its health benefits. Gillian, when our paths cross for real, I hope to enjoy a giant buttery steak with you while we enthusiastically discuss just how much we love this way of life.

To the recipe testers who volunteered their time to test my recipes at their own expense, your role is so critical when creating a good cookbook: Angie, Cindy, Heino, Gabby, Joanita, Julie, Kimmy and Jay, Pippa, Stella and Tanya – thank you for your insight and feedback.

To the readers of *Keto Kitchen*: your support and praise humbled me to the core, and I was thrilled to see your creations on social media. Your comments continue to warm my heart and bring a little lump to my throat.

To my colleagues at The Fat Duck, both past and present: I love you all. You have shaped the way I think about food.

Lastly, to my darling Mark... some may say you are a lucky man being married to someone who experiments and creates different and exciting meals every night, but this is simply not true: I am the lucky one! Your peppered lamb ribs and 'Mark's famous chicken' are still my favourite things to eat, and it's not because those are the nights I can put my feet up – it's because I can taste the love you put into them. I love you too xxx.

Monya